ACTIVISM IS
MEDICINE

ACTIVISM IS MEDICINE

Health and Relevance for
the Human Animal

FRANK FORENCICH

ISBN (print): 978-0-9723358-1-2

ISBN: (ebook): 978-0-9723358-2-9

Published by Exuberant Animal, Bend, Oregon

HUMANANIMAL.EARTH

ACTIVISMISMEDICINE.NET

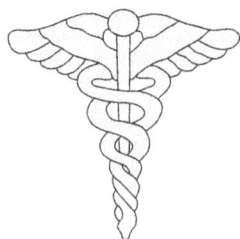

Warning:

*Before beginning a program of inactivism
or disengagement, see your doctor.*

CONTENTS

PREFACE

Doing nothing is an extremist position.

Dr. Charlie Gardner
conservation biologist

When I travel the world of activism and engagement, people sometimes ask "When did you first become radicalized?" Or to put it another way, How did you come to your extremist perspective? Were you always this way, or was there a pivotal event that changed your world view? Why are you so different from other, normal people?

I listen politely, but before long I become confused. It sounds like maybe I'm being judged as an outlier, a troublemaker, or someone who's camped out on the lunatic fringe. Maybe it's a compliment or maybe I'm being lumped in with the crazies. These days, it's hard to tell.

The problem is that when it comes to the word *radical*, there are just too many definitions in play. Sometimes it means "going to the root of things," but it also suggests extreme beliefs, especially the destruction of established social and cultural norms. And it can even mean excellence, as in "your moves that climb were totally rad, dude."

But speaking for myself, I'm not at all sure that the word fits, at least not in the way that most people understand it. Instead, I've lived some powerful experiences that have given me insight into the state of the planet and the role that humans might play. Along the way, I've come to realize that my personal philosophy is not radical at all, but deeply conservative. In fact, interviewers might do better to ask "When did you first become conservatized?"

To answer *that* question, my journey began decades ago in the Boy Scouts, when I first learned to pay attention to the natural world. I got comfortable in the mountains and in turn, my sense of biophilia began to grow. But then I read Paul Ehrlich's 1971 book *The Population Bomb* and got my first glimpse of a looming, dysfunctional future. A few years later I flew over the Pacific Northwest in a small aircraft and witnessed the vast clear-cuts that scarred every mountain and valley, a checkerboard of habitat destruction as far as I could see.

Next up was the program in human biology at Stanford, a long apprenticeship in the martial arts, and a year in massage school, all of which intensified my curiosity about the history and function of the human body, especially in a historical context. Along the way, I saw the gruesome photos of the Alberta Tar Sands project and followed the 2016 pipeline protests at Standing Rock. I witnessed the decimation of shark populations in the restaurants of Hong Kong. I saw my childhood bioregion destroyed by development; rich orchards and green spaces obliterated by McMansions, relentless commerce, and outrageous affluence.

Trying to make sense of it all, I read every green book I could get my hands on: *The Green History of the World*,

Overshoot, Sand County Almanac, Silent Spring, Green Rage, The End of Nature, The Voice of the Earth, and of course, *The Monkey Wrench Gang.* I followed the careers of writers and activists around the world: Henry David Thoreau, Rachel Carson, Aldo Leopold, Dave Foreman, Edward Abbey, Theodore Roszak, E.O. Wilson, Paul Watson, Derrick Jensen, Greta Thunberg, and a host of others. I read deeply about the world views of native and indigenous people around the world and I even traveled to Africa to study our ancestral homeland where I spent some time with the Hadza bushmen.

Was I radicalized by these experiences? Not in the way you might think. Ultimately, I began to realize that the true radicals on this planet are those who are destroying the natural world—the only life support system in the known universe. Fossil fuel executives are radical. Corporations that practice strip mining, sea floor mining, deforestation and industrial-scale fish harvesting are radical. Politicians who refuse to deal with climate chaos and extinction; anyone who sides with the continued destruction of the biosphere—these are the true extremists of our age.

In contrast, the defenders of our planet are best described as conservatives and conservationists. Those who protest, those who get in the way, those who speak out and disrupt the radical acts of industrial-scale violence, inconvenient people who aren't afraid to speak up—these people are doing essential, courageous, creative, and inspirational work. They are agents of nature, defending herself.

And while I may be deeply conservative in my views, I'm also angry, which is say, my hair is on fire. Everything I hold dear is being systematically destroyed by greed, ignorance, and bad actors. I'm outraged that defenders of the Earth are being targeted for prosecution and like many, I'm suffering my share of grief, anxiety, and pain. As someone who identifies deeply with the natural world, I feel the destruction as a direct, traumatizing assault on my body and my spirit. My heart is breaking.

This is why I write. This is why I speak. This is why I need the medicine. And so my friend, this book is dedicated to the conservatives among us: the biophiliacs, the disruptors, and the creators. If your hair is on fire and you need the medicine, this book is for you.

PREDICAMENT

Anything else you're interested in is not going to happen if you can't breathe the air and drink the water. Don't sit this one out. Do something. You are by accident of fate alive at an absolutely critical moment in the history of our planet.

Carl Sagan

It's worse than you think.
It's bigger than you think.

It's more catastrophic, persistent, and consequential than you think. And it's happening way, way faster than you think.

The human animal—and the rest of life on earth—is in serious trouble. Whatever your assessment of the human predicament at this moment in history, conditions are in fact more extreme than most people realize. As David Wallace-Wells put it in his 2019 book *The Uninhabitable Earth*, "No matter how well-informed you are, you are surely not alarmed enough."

No matter who you are or your role in the world, the planet is now the elephant in the room. Soft language calls it "climate change," but it's actually an "everything change." It's a climate, ecological, and spiritual emergency, marked by abrupt and possibly irreversible transformation of Earth systems. All the scientific fire alarms are going off. As Greta Thunberg puts it, "The house is on fire." (And the arsonists are in charge.)

Climate gets most of our attention as well it should, but this is actually a full-spectrum, 3-dimensional crisis, a wicked cluster of wicked problems. Call it what you will: a polycrisis, a permacrisis, a metacrisis, a hyperthreat, the Anthropocene, the Pyrocene, a mass extinction event, the Age of Consequences, or Planetary Endgame. But no matter what we call it, the emergency is both broad and deep. It's a public health crisis, a cultural crisis, a psycho-spiritual crisis, a moral crisis, a relational crisis, and a crisis of our collective imagination. All our systems are stretched to the limit: agriculture, transportation, energy, materials, medicine, education, government, human nervous systems, and the human psyche itself. If the biosphere was a human body, we'd say that it's experiencing a multi-organ failure.

Without question, the state of the planet is the alpha crisis of our age and the most consequential challenge in the history of humanity. As author Naomi Klein has put it "When your life support system is threatened, all other problems fit inside that problem." In other words, every other issue is secondary. When there's a gaping hole in your lifeboat, the priority is—or should be—obvious.

A quick sampling of actual headlines from 2023 tells the story:

Earth's hottest day in at least 125,000 years

UN Secretary General Warns Fossil Fuels "incompatible with human survival"

Mutilating the tree of life: Wildlife loss accelerating, scientists warn

Earth is outside its 'safe operating space for humanity' on most key measurements, study says

Ecosystems will collapse within a human lifespan, warns a new study

Physicists predict Earth will become a chaotic world, with dire consequences

Climate Crisis Is on Track to Push One-Third of Humanity Out of Its Most Livable Environment

Food shortages and wars expected as world warms

UN Warns Earth 'firmly on track toward an unlivable world'

Even Pope Francis understands the gravity of the situation. In a statement released in October 2023, the pontiff stressed the irreversible damage under way to the planet and its people, adding that the world's poor and most vulnerable were paying the highest price. As he put it, we live on a "suffering planet" that "may be nearing a breaking point."

The stakes couldn't possibly be higher. We risk losing everything we hold dear—not just habitable bioregions and loved ones, but all the hard-won fruits of civilization. The sheer magnitude of suffering on this planet is poised to dwarf anything we've experienced in human history. Widespread famine and food insecurity are likely, extreme social conflict, rising inequality and chaos, and break downs in health and social support systems around the world. And the clock isn't just ticking, it's screaming in our ears and our faces, demanding that we take this thing seriously *now*.

LIFE IN THE QUAGMIRE

But bad as it is, our predicament is about a lot more than atmospheric physics or ecosystem biology. It also poses an epic, potentially catastrophic challenge to human consciousness, attention and mental-spiritual health. In fact, a substantial proportion of humanity has at least one foot in the mental health quagmire already: depression, anxiety, insomnia, stress-related disorders, social dysfunction, distraction, addiction, and identity crises. We often treat these afflictions as distinct, isolated disorders, but they're really part of a larger whole—the human struggle with adaptation in a monstrously challenging, and rapidly disintegrating world.

A perfect storm of stress, anxiety, and trauma is surging through the collective unconscious of humanity. Fear and hyper-vigilance are widespread, amplified by always-on media and a hockey-stick acceleration of novelty, innovation and radical change. Familiar forms of trauma are challenging enough, but today we're plagued by entirely new set of afflictions, variously described as eco-anxiety, eco-distress, climate anxiety, collapse anxiety, and extinction grief, all of which are rising in prevalence and intensity around the world, especially in young people. To put it simply, many of us don't trust the future, or even the present for that matter.

Not only are people suffering, so too are non-human animals and habitats around the world. And inevitably, humans feel this pain as well. As the ecopsychologist Theodore Roszak put it, "The Earth hurts and we hurt with it." The great psychologist Carl Jung made a similar observation in *The Earth Has a Soul*: "Man feels himself isolated in the cosmos. He is no longer involved in nature and has lost his emotional participation in natural events." Or, as Aldo Leopold famously put it in *A Sand County Almanac*, "One of the penalties of an ecological education is that one lives alone in a world of wounds."

Numerous studies confirm an epidemic of loneliness, even among people who are superficially connected. And not surprisingly, "deaths of despair"—including suicide and deaths related to substance abuse—are on the rise. It's no wonder that the prevalence of addiction is increasing around the world. As professor Bruce Alexander put it in his 2010 book *The Globalization of Addiction* "Globalization of free-market society has produced an unprecedented, worldwide collapse of psychosocial integration."

Even worse, we're caught up in what professor John Vervaeke calls a "crisis of meaning." To put it simply, our stories no longer work. We're caught between two equally untenable narratives about who we are and where we might be going. On one hand is the dominant, preposterous story of human supremacy: *Homo sapiens* is the greatest animal ever to walk the Earth; we are the sole protagonist in this drama and nature is nothing more than a supporting cast. On the other hand is an emerging shadow narrative: Humans are the most dangerous animal in the history of life. We are the cancer, the virus, the pathogen, the asteroid—nothing but a failed biological experiment and an evolutionary dead-end.

Vervaeke describes our meaning crisis in stark terms:

> It's more and more pervasive throughout our lives and there's a sense of drowning in an ocean of bullshit. People are feeling disconnected from themselves, from each other, from the world, and from a viable and foreseeable future.

All of which adds up to a monstrous psycho-spiritual crisis for the human animal. Holocaust survivor Viktor Frankl wrote about the "existential vacuum" that pervades the modern world, a condition that The American Psychological Association defines as "the inability to find or create meaning in life, leading to feelings of emptiness, alienation, futility, and aimlessness." And so the questions nag, especially as we enter the middle years of our lives. "How is my life meaningful? Am I relevant? Does my life even matter? Is there even a path? Is there a meaningful way to live that's relevant and consistent with ecological reality? Many of us are beginning to doubt it all.

Around the world, people are looking for support, secure attachment and a coherent explanation of our place in the world and increasingly, we seek out therapy. It's a wise move, but the demand is immense and growing. Most therapists are booked out months in advance and even if we're lucky enough to find a sensitive ear, it's not altogether clear that today's therapists know what to do in the face of planetary-level trauma. Our understanding of neuroscience is impressive and our technological expertise undeniable, but we're failing to develop and nurture the whole human animal.

As a result, most of Earth's human population is suffering. Some of us are stunned into a state of passivity and inaction, others are lulled into a kind of sleep-walking acceptance of abnormality and alienation. Lost in an incoherent world that seems hell-bent on its destruction, most of us are hanging on by our fingernails.

THE CASE FOR ACTIVISM

All of which brings us to this book and the obvious question: How is it that we're talking about activism and medicine, two domains that might well seem to have nothing whatsoever to do with one another? Medicine is all about disease, infection, antibiotics, physical exams, diagnosis, and treatment. Activism is all about politics, legislation, organizing, fundraising, messaging, and civil disobedience. To the casual observer, they look like two completely different challenges, with miles of empty space between them. But what if we're wrong about all of this? What if activism is actually integral to health itself?

On the face of it, it might well seem that political activism doesn't offer any of the familiar challenges we've come to associate with promoting good health—holding up a sign on a street corner doesn't burn many calories, filing a petition or writing a letter doesn't build muscle. Go to a conference, write a book, testify in front of a committee, get arrested—these things sound stressful and maybe even health-negative. Who ever heard of someone going into activism intentionally as a health practice?

But what if activism is bigger and more powerful than we realize? What if there are genuine health benefits that

come with engagement? Might it be true that by focusing our efforts on creating change, we also improve the
state of our minds and bodies? Could activism actually
make us stronger? What if activism actually nourishes us
with vital understandings and experiences? Wouldn't that
change everything?

A PATH, A PRACTICE, A WAY

Naturally, all of this depends on how we do it. Not just
any kind of activism will have a therapeutic effect on the
human animal and in fact, it's easy to imagine plenty of
actions that would take our health down the wrong path.
Simply showing up with a banner and an attitude isn't going to do much for your body or the world for that matter.
No, to make this work, we've got to practice our activism
in a particular way, with the right attention and intention,
and that's the beauty of it. This is far more than impulsive
reaction to particular issues or injustices, this is a practice,
a path, and a way to relate to the world and life as a whole.

In conventional circles, most people think of activism—
if they think of it at all—as an isolated, occasional endeav-
or for highly-motivated, passionate or angry people. It's
hard work, often frustrating, exhausting, and stressful.
The effort may well be laudable and even inspiring on
some level, but it's not for normal, regular people.

In contrast, this book takes a more expansive view. That
is, activism is for everyone, no matter their background,
resources or capabilities. It's about politics to be sure, but
it's also about how we choose to live. It's about power,
strategy and tactics, but it's really about how we relate to
the world at large. It's about the decisions we make, the

perspectives we hold, the language we use, the things that we buy and the things we create. It's about the totality of our lives, both the inner and the outer game of change. And most of all, it's about how we show up.

RESISTANCE IS FERTILE

The fascinating thing about activism is that—like physical exercise—it's both a sign of health and a pathway to health. People with vitality are more likely to engage with the world, both with vigorous physical movement and efforts to drive social and cultural change. Likewise, people who engage are likely to improve their health along the way. For the healthy human animal, activism is proof of life, wildness, vitality, and even sanity. It gives us credibility as healthy, robust wild animals and should be viewed as part of a regular health practice.

Unfortunately, we're up against some powerful cultural baggage. In the popular imagination, activism sounds like a burden, a stressor and a major inconvenience. Why should I get involved political and social change? Why should I spend my time and expose myself to opposition, adversity and uncertainty, not to mention the possibility of jail time or worse? After all, you probably aren't going to get paid for your efforts and you'll have to expose yourself to a public that doesn't appreciate your work or even worse, attacks your beliefs and your legitimacy. It might even be physically dangerous. On the face of it, the whole thing sounds like a raw deal.

The problem is that we forget the positives, or to be more precise, we've never actually heard about the positives in the first place. To be sure, there's always going to be plenty of stress and frustration in the process of creating social change, but activism also gives back in some meaningful and exciting ways. Taking responsibility for the state of the world will sometimes feel like a burden, but it's also an incredibly meaningful adventure that makes our lives more complete. As activists in Extinction Rebellion have put it, *resistance is fertile.*

As we'll see, the primary value of activism lies in its integrating effect on the human animal. The practice is very much akin to vigorous physical movement, otherwise known as exercise. When we act intentionally and take risks, particularly in the face of ambiguity and uncertainty, we call on the body-mind-spirit to gather its resources into a single, cohesive effort. This integrating effect can be powerfully health-positive, especially when we operate in the sweet spot of stress. A solid body of work in medical research shows that having a sense of meaning and purpose in life is associated with positive health outcomes. In other words, it's clinically significant.

But activism is more than just a way to change the world; it's also a powerful way to learn and know the world. Every time we go outside our comfort zone and engage in action, we grow. Every time we push back against entrenched power, we discover something new about law, policy and government. We learn about the history of our people, our institutions and our culture. We learn about complex systems and most importantly, we learn about human behavior, stress, psychology and inclinations. We learn about the dynamics of obedience, groupthink, persuasion and influence. We learn about our personal values, our identity, our character, and our performance under pressure. All of which amounts to some precious life lessons and skill development—education that would be impossible via conventional textbooks and classroom lectures.

Activism also sparks our creativity. When faced with overwhelming opposition and complexity, improv is essential. Every situation is different and rarely do we have an established play book to guide us. Direct confrontation often fails and we're forced to try new approaches including indirect, lateral moves and artistic workarounds; sometimes we just have to make things up on the fly. This process is powerfully stimulating for individual and group creativity and can even be incredibly fun.

Likewise, activism can be a party. All the best actions come about through intensive collaboration, planning, problem-solving and support, all of which puts us in contact with interesting, creative and courageous people. In the process, we often experience a powerful sense of belonging and a realization that "these are my people."

The beauty of this social effort is that it gets us out of our isolated selves and into the world. As most of us have heard or discovered the hard way, too much isolation leads to all manner of discontent, anxiety, and psycho-spiritual dysfunction. Activism puts us in contact with one another and in the process, serves as a powerful antidote to the narcissism and loneliness of our age.

A related benefit comes with what psychologists call our sense of "mattering." All people have a deep and compelling need to feel that their existence is important in some way. We want to feel valued and we want to add value to the world around us. Research suggests that people who feel valued experience more self-compassion, relationship satisfaction, and greater belief in their capacity to achieve their goals. Conversely, lack of mattering is associated with burnout, self-criticism, anxiety, depression, aggression and increased risk of suicide. The beauty of activism is that it helps to fill this basic human need; start contributing to a cause or an issue and it won't be long before you'll feel like you're part of something significant.

Along the way, we might even come to the conclusion that activism is a form of therapy. Naturally, success will lie in the details, but done properly, it makes sense to say that activism can have a healing effect on the human animal, especially in the way it promotes focus and intentional, conscious engagement. Activism sharpens our attention and forces us to engage with greater awareness. Even better, it also puts us in contact with supportive, caring communities. Above all, activism gives us an enhanced sense of meaning and relevance in the world. Win or lose, we become part of something important, something larger than ourselves.

HOW TO SHOW UP

Perhaps the greatest benefit of activism is that it teaches us how to show up in our lives and in the world at large. In this sense, it's really part of a long human tradition that we see in religion, craft, athletics, therapy and counseling, even the professions. Across all these pursuits, there's specialized knowledge and skills to be mastered, but even more to the point, there's a psycho-physical presence that must be cultivated and nurtured. This is the true heart of the experience.

Just imagine participating in a high-pressure action or engagement—a protest, a big meeting or a public presentation. There's going to be pressure, opposition, and surprises along the way; it's hard to know how unpredictable humans are going to respond to your actions. To make it work, you've got to show up with a balanced psycho-physical presence, otherwise known as equipoise. You'll want to be as attentive, curious, flexible, sincere, and integrated as possible. In the process you'll make errors and sometimes you'll even show up with the wrong attitude, but with practice, you'll get better at bringing your best game to the engagement. This alone—completely independent of any particular win or lose outcome—is reason enough to get involved.

For many, this approach will sound and feel unfamiliar, even alien. Living in our conventional, rewards-based culture, we tend to be highly focused on outcomes. Almost from birth, we've been systematically trained to pursue good grades, awards, bonuses, and all manner of perks in the worlds of education, career, and commerce. As educator Alfie Kohn put it in *Punished by Rewards*, modern culture tells us "Do this and you'll get that." Given this conditioning, it's no surprise to find a similar orientation in the world of activism; there's work to be done, so we focus on outcomes and if we fail to create the changes we seek, we're likely to become depressed and maybe even drop out of engagement entirely.

A better perspective is to view the activist experience as *autotelic*, something with intrinsic value, completely independent of any particular outcome. Activism is simply good for us, full stop. Act with passion, creativity, and integrity and you'll develop more of the same. Obviously, we're looking for some measure of effectiveness along the way and we might well say that the natural world very much needs us to succeed, but it's also essential that we recognize the inherent value in the doing. Objectives and destinations *are* important, but the journey is what really matters. And if the journey looks valuable and interesting, more people are likely to join in.

ABOUT THIS BOOK

As you'll see, this is a book about creating a life of engagement, meaning and relevance. It describes the overwhelming and sometimes unbearable nature of our predicament, but it also offers a surprisingly positive vision for the human animal. It's often said that "action is the antidote to despair," but it's even more than that. Action—and the orientation behind it—has a powerful focusing effect and is massively therapeutic for the entire organism and sometimes even the world around it. Done properly, with forethought and care, activism can make you a stronger and more effective person.

In essence, this book is about the way that humans respond in their encounter with The Knowledge, the realization that the biosphere is in mortal danger. Some of us will ignore the call and carry on as if nothing is amiss, while some will rise to the occasion with passion and intensity in pursuit of systemic change.

Obviously, this book is a call to action, but even more to the point, it's a call to creativity. Our predicament is daunting and all of us are susceptible to resignation, cynicism, and despair. The challenge is to take that burden and turn it into something interesting, something meaningful, maybe even something beautiful. Start showing up for the future and you'll wind up feeling a whole lot better in the process.

ENCOUNTER

Do not look away.

Roger Hallam
co-founder of Extinction Rebellion

We start our journey as educational virgins, knowing nothing of atmospheres, biospheres, carbon pollution, species extinctions, corporate dominance of society or the destructive beliefs of human supremacy. Protected from danger in infancy and childhood, our parents and teachers worked to keep us safe from unpleasant realities and insulate us from the hostilities of the larger world.

As well they should. This comforting protection is vital to the development of the young animal and must be supported by society as a whole. Children who are well-protected grow up stronger, healthier and more resilient; we need more of this. But sooner or later, there comes a reckoning. At some point, the comforting embrace of childhood must give way to something more realistic. Slowly or suddenly, it begins to dawn on us that dangers, adversities, pain and suffering are real. We learn that life can hurt us.

Making a successful transition into adulthood requires that we integrate and metabolize these realizations into our psyche, into some kind of functional relationship with the world at large. If the young human animal can absorb these inconvenient truths about the world without becoming terrified or numb, she'll have a chance at success.

The process is psychological, but it's also biological, driven in large measure by the autonomic nervous system, the ancient regulatory wiring that lies deep within the body. Most of us have heard the basic description of the two branches by now: one devoted to emergency physical action (fight-flight), the other to healing and rejuvenation (rest-and-digest or feed-and-breed).

Likewise, most of us have heard that chronic activation of the fight-flight system is corrosive to our health, our performance and our longevity. The trick for healthy and functional living is to stay in a relaxed, rest-and-digest state as much as possible; don't activate the stress response unless you really need it.

The autonomic system is incredibly powerful in determining our health and performance over the course of our lives, but it's far more than just a bunch of squishy neurons, wires and circuitry. The autonomic is guided by incredibly sophisticated brain structures that interpret experiences and surroundings, directing the system to go in one direction or the other. In essence, the brain makes a judgment call on danger and sends its interpretation into the body where the autonomic system can take action or rest and heal up.

For the autonomic, the first priority is always survival; the prime directive is to sense danger and keep us safe. In effect, the system asks a simple, primal question in every minute of every day: "Is my world friendly?" If the answer is "no" we go on alert and start taking protective action. If the answer is "yes," we start rebuilding tissue and putting the body back together. And if the answer is an ambiguous "I'm not sure," the body struggles to find its psycho-physical equilibrium. But in any case, all of this neural activity and response hinges on perception, interpretation, story and meaning.

For the young child in a healthy environment, the answer to the "friendly question" is usually a resounding "yes." Parents give warmth, love and attention and the child feels felt; she knows that people are paying attention and taking care of her needs. She has yet to understand much about the world, but it *feels* safe and comforting. In turn, she can devote her resources to growth, development, play and learning. All is well.

But a reckoning comes soon enough. We try to walk, take a few steps, fall down and scrape our knees. In that instant, we begin to realize that the world isn't always friendly, but never fear, comforting adults step in to patch us up and help us get back on our feet. The cuts and bruises heal and we're free to go back to the playground.

Later, our awareness grows and we begin to realize that the unfriendly forces are bigger and more powerful than we'd imagined. Things can hurt us in tragic and traumatic ways that no Band-Aid can fix. Animals, vehicles, and even the people close to us can inflict intense pain on our bodies and minds. Danger lurks and the world begins to feel complex, ambiguous and unpredictable. Once again, our elders try to help us feel safe, but we also learn to build defenses of our own: cognitive, physical, social, financial, and spiritual. It's good and important work, and many of us eventually learn how to navigate a world that's both friendly and unfriendly.

RUDE AWAKENINGS

All of which is familiar territory in our individual human experience, but today there's a unique challenge looming—our encounter with The Knowledge, the fact that the natural world is in mortal danger and that we might not have a functional future to look forward to. This inspires a new kind of fear and an unprecedented level of anxiety in the human animal—a fresh hell you might say.

To put it in terms our prehistoric ancestors could understand, imagine that you're living in a camp on the savanna of East Africa, some 100,000 years ago. On a typical day you might encounter a handful of carnivores prowling the outskirts of your territory, but you've co-evolved with these animals and your people have developed a sophisticated understanding of their behavior—knowledge that's embedded in your oral tradition. The carnivores are still dangerous and must be respected, but if you pay attention and listen to the guidance of your elders, you can usually avoid the worst of it.

But today the situation has escalated radically and now it feels as if thousands of carnivores are poised to attack our camp and terrorize the entire planet at any moment. We have no history with this predicament and our traditions tell us nothing about how to adapt. Even worse, some of our elders are either denying the reality of the carnivores outright or are actively facilitating their behavior. In the long history of the human animal, nothing like this has ever happened and the autonomic nervous system has no idea how to respond.

For some, this realization will come about as a traumatic shock, a shattering insight that disrupts our lives and demands our attention. Bright young students read and hear about ecocide, carrying capacity, overshoot, and the relentless trauma that industrial society continues to inflict on the natural world. They grasp the enormity of the challenge and do their best to cope, but the answers are unsatisfying at best. For others, the understanding comes incrementally as a steady drip of bad news and partial awakenings that wear down our defenses and leave us naked before the ecological truth. We try our best to escape, but the facts follow us around wherever we go and eventually, we're forced to take reality seriously. Or not.

For those who do choose to pay attention, the first rude awakening is the simple realization that scientists have been telling the truth for decades and continue to do so. Errors are always possible, but the method includes robust corrective mechanisms that move our understanding ever closer to an accurate description of reality. In short, science does what it claims to do; we can trust its findings.

So consider these crystal-clear warnings and clarion calls to action: Rachel Carson's 1962 *Silent Spring*, the 1972 report *Limits to Growth*, William Catton's 1982 *Overshoot: The Ecological Basis of Revolutionary Change*, Carl Sagan's 1985 testimony to Congress, James Hansen's 1988 testimony to Congress, Bill McKibben's 1989 *The End of Nature*, E.O. Wilson's 1992 *The Diversity of Life*, Al Gore's 2006 documentary *An Inconvenient Truth*, and the 2015 Paris Agreement. It's not as if we haven't been warned.

To sum up the scientific findings...

- The climate crisis is real.

- The biodiversity and extinction crisis is real.

- Widespread habitat destruction is real.

- Marine heat waves and ocean acidification are real.

- Melting glaciers, thawing permafrost and catastrophic methane emissions are real.

- Deforestation, desertification and freshwater depletion are real.

- Global light pollution and noise pollution are real.

- Fertilizer runoff and marine dead zones are real.

- Rising sea levels and extreme weather events are real.

All these facts have nothing to do with belief, faith or religion by the way. A reporter asks "Do you believe in climate change?" Do you believe in our ecological crisis, the depletion of biodiversity, deforestation, desertification or the exploitation of the oceans?

These are bad questions that must be re-framed, over and over again. None of this is a matter of belief—it's a matter of understanding. This is about hard scientific reality and, as some atmospheric scientists have put it, "physics doesn't care what you believe."

NON-LINEAR CHANGE

If this was the extent of our reckoning, that would be plenty bad enough, but the next rude awakening comes with our understanding of non-linear change in dynamic natural systems. In short, our atmosphere and biosphere can change almost in an instant. Positive feedback amplifies the process; once a threshold or tipping point is crossed, change begins to accelerate dramatically and at this point, things happen really fast.

Most obviously, this is what we see in today's atmosphere, a highly dynamic system that is now undergoing accelerating transformation as numerous thresholds are crossed. To cite just one example: when Arctic sea ice melts, darker water is exposed, absorbing more heat and in turn, increasing the rate of global heating and melting yet more ice. And as heat increases, permafrost in the Arctic also melts, releasing methane—a potent greenhouse gas—which heats the atmosphere further. In other words, the hotter it gets, the faster the warming.

This atmospheric instability is very real and extremely consequential. In fact, earlier climate models were too conservative: changes to the atmosphere and biosphere are happening much faster than anticipated. The Intergovernmental Panel on Climate Change has called this "the most rapid environmental change in planetary history." When we cross the threshold of 1.5 degrees of atmospheric warming, 2, 3, and 4 degrees won't be far behind. And if these sound like small numbers, don't be fooled. All are harbingers of mass extinction, migration, famine, and catastrophic, non-linear social chaos. Millions of people will likely die in coming decades. Not a pretty picture.

BIG CAPITALISM

But these rude awakenings—disturbing as they are—are just the beginning of our reckoning. For those who care to look, another shock comes with the realization that our neoliberal economic system is rapidly destroying the habitability of our planet. In short, big-money capitalism is starting to look like a failed concept, if not an outright criminal enterprise.

The problem is that, in essence, the modern corporation is nothing more than a mindless legal machine for generating profit for executives and shareholders. The formula is simple: internalize profit and externalize cost. Or to put it another way, privatize the gains and socialize the loses. Whenever possible, shift the burden of externalities (pollution, noise, disease) onto the community and let the people handle it. Capture the policy making process with brute force lobbying, starve the health and human services sector, and reap the bounty along the way. In 2023, a Greenpeace billboard captured the corporate mindset perfectly—against a vivid backdrop of raging wildfires in Greece, the Shell corporation declares "Our profit, your loss."

Even worse, the modern corporation enjoys and profits by its legal personhood status, similar to that enjoyed by individual people. In turn, this begs the obvious question: How can it be that natural, living entities of our planet have essentially no rights, but corporations do? In the eyes of the law, forests, rivers, lakes, oceans, marshlands, and species are regarded as nothing more than inert objects, while corporations are given nearly free reign. This is beginning to change with the growing rights of nature movement, but there's still a long way to go.

In essence, industrial capitalism regards the natural world as an infinite resource with no intrinsic value, there for the taking without limit. Social and ecological consequences are irrelevant to the operation of the machine. In its relentless drive for profit, the mechanism turns communities—both human and non-human—into commodities. This extraction ideology has no built-in end point and actively resists any regulatory process that might keep it in check. If this same kind of process existed within a human body, we'd call it neoplastic or cancerous. If it was part of a machine, a vehicle, or an aircraft, engineers would quickly develop countermeasures to keep the process from spiraling out of control.

The problem is the corporate mechanism itself, but even worse, it's also a matter of brazen, naked criminality at the top. It's now widely understood that fossil fuel companies knew full well the destructive effects of their products as far back as the 1980's and not only persisted with business as usual, but actively blocked efforts at mitigation.

Without question, this is criminal behavior of the highest order, a prime example of ecocide. In fact, activist Bill McKibben and others have described it as the most egregious crime in human history. Roger Hallam, founder of Extinction Rebellion, has called it out as "murder by the elite."

Likewise, more and more people are talking about intergenerational genocide perpetrated by fossil fuel corporations, while others describe the near-term future as a "fossil-fueled Holocaust." And if this sounds hyperbolic, think again. In all likelihood, far more people are going to die in coming decades than in all the concentration camps in Germany. By destroying the habitability of entire bioregions, we're effectively destroying the people who live there. In other words, ecocide *is* genocide.

BIG INEQUALITY

All of which leads to yet another rude awakening, namely the staggering levels of social and economic inequality, most notably the imperialism by the global North over the global South. The gap between rich and poor is not only immense but is poised to grow ever larger as environmental pressures increase around the world. To a large extent, the rich can temporarily buffer themselves against the consequences of the climate crisis, but the poor can only suffer.

Not only does the North exploit labor and resources of the South, it also uses the South as a dumping ground for the byproducts of industrial activity. The injustice is stark: the people least responsible for climate-wrecking emissions are now suffering the lion's share of the consequences. All of which is best described as a reverse Robin Hood program, robbing from the poor and giving to the rich. In effect, rapacious corporations, in cooperation with big government, have devised a wealth pump that sucks profit upwards while it drives stress hormones and pollution downwards.

INDUSTRIAL AGRICULTURE

Not only does big corporate power drive social inequality, it also drives an agricultural system that is breathtaking in its destructiveness. Look closely at the back story of modern food production and you'll see a vast, globalized system built on fossil fuels, pesticides, herbicides, vanishing groundwater, and plastic packaging–all of it devoted not to human nourishment, but to corporate profit.

Few people realize the full extent of the damage, but it's essential to recognize the fact that modern agriculture is itself a form of habitat destruction. By planting monocultures and protecting them from natural change, industrial agriculture effectively destroys biodiversity. Meat production is by far the biggest offender, deforesting large tracts of land to grow food for cattle, while palm oil production is responsible for deforesting immense regions of Malaysia and Indonesia. Without question, these are some of the most egregious, habitat-destroying practices on the planet today.

But that's just the beginning. Modern ultra-processed food-like-substances also have a devastating effect on the human body. We've all heard a good deal about the familiar afflictions of diabetes and obesity, but modern agricultural practices also contribute to drastic modifications to the gut microbiome, with ripple effects that reach all the way to the brain and nervous systems. Practitioners in the emerging field of nutritional psychiatry point to impaired cognitive function and neuro-behavioral disorders that can be traced back to our alien, adulterated food supply.

In short, our food system is built on the suffering, not just of the animals that are consumed by humans, but of all the animals that are rendered homeless by our relentless drive for calories, protein, beef, and palm oil. The rude awakening comes with almost every meal: nearly every bite of food we eat is ecologically or ethically compromised, or more likely, both.

CULTURE SHOCK

Big corporate power is obviously a toxic, often criminal

enterprise that threatens to destroy our future, but there are even more rude awakenings in store—in particular, the realization that the standard narrative of modern culture is itself a recipe for catastrophe. To put it another way, the climate crisis is about a lot more than atmospheric physics. It's a food crisis, a water crisis, a health crisis, and a humanitarian crisis, but even more than all that, it's a cultural-relational-spiritual crisis.

Looking closer, we see a cluster of culturally sanctioned ideas and assumptions that move us ever closer to collapse as they pull us deeper into the mental health quagmire. The problem begins with a rejection of the historically normal indigenous, kin-centric orientation, replaced by a human-centered, anthropocentric world view, sometimes described as *anthropofascist*.

As conventional culture sees it, humans are superior to all other species and the rules of nature simply don't apply. The plants, animals, and microorganisms of the planet may be interdependent, but humans are—by our own declaration—independent. The circle of life has now been replaced by a fantasy pyramid, with Western humanity claiming the alpha position. And in this world, almost nothing—with the exception of profit—is sacred.

All of which sounds suspiciously like the "Dark Triad" of narcissism, Machiavellianism, and psychopathy that's been observed by psychologists in the domain of human relationships. If industrial civilization was a person, it would display all the hallmarks of the disorder, especially the absence of empathy and remorse. To put it simply, "It's all about me, I am willing to hurt you for my gain, and I don't care how you feel." Is it any wonder that people raised in such a culture exhibit similar traits?

Closely related is the popular belief in the myth of progress—the assumption that the human condition inevitably evolves towards perfection, a belief that eco-theologian Michael Dowd called "the secular religion of perpetual progress." This doctrine implies that everything that came before the present moment is by definition inferior. In other words, our ancestors were nothing more than brutish hunters with primitive, childish ideas about the world. This intellectual imperialism tells us that there's only one way to understand the world, and we know what it is. Ancient and indigenous forms of knowing, built up methodically over millennia are simply irrelevant.

At the same time, we see the intensification of the ego and a relentless focus on the individual, a state that David Brooks of the New York Times calls "the Big Me." As he sees it, modern society has suffered an erosion in moral education and sensitivity over the last century, now replaced by a growing and highly commercialized focus on the self. In short, young people are now growing up in a "morally inarticulate, self-referential world."

Wider circles of society and habitat are ignored as individuals double down on their personal desires and interests. Today, it's not just acceptable to be self-focused and narcissistic, it's actually considered virtuous. In our highly competitive achievement culture, personal branding and self-promotion are celebrated as vital pathways to success. All of which leads to a world of toxic individualism where it's "every man for himself, every woman for herself."

In this context, it's no surprise to find that individual suffering is often framed as nothing more than just that. It's simply an affliction of the isolated human body and mind, completely independent of surrounding forces. If you're suffering from anxiety or depression in your school or workplace, you need to meditate, build your personal resilience and practice personal self-help. Little or nothing is said about the negative influences of setting, context, predicament, or large scale systems. Little or nothing is said about the need for activism or system change. If you're suffering, that's *your* problem.

For those of us living inside this world, these ideas might well seem familiar, and therefore normal, but native people see our modern orientation as nothing less than a psycho-spiritual illness. *Wetiko* is an Algonquin word for a cannibalistic spirit that is driven by greed, excess, and selfish consumption. It deludes its host into believing that consuming the life-force of others (including animals and other forms of life) is a logical and morally upright way to live.

Sometimes called "the white man's disease," *wetiko* short-circuits the individual's ability to see herself as an enmeshed and interdependent part of a balanced environment and raises the self-serving ego to supremacy. In its embrace of nature-human separation, its blatant disregard for the welfare of other creatures, and the rejection of the natural world as a whole, it's not much of an exaggeration to describe modern society as a "death culture."

In simpler times, human culture served a distinct survival purpose, even acting as a psycho-spiritual womb for developing children and adults under stress. Stories and rituals gave us a sense of security and helped us navigate the challenges of survival. Even more importantly, culture gave us an explanation, a reason for our existence that put our minds at ease. In a very real sense, culture was a true life-support system.

But today, the situation is radically reversed. Not only does modern culture fail to give us a coherent, plausible explanation for our existence and a purpose for living, it actually deepens our alienation and suffering. No longer does it help us survive; it's actually anti-functional and ecocidal. We might even go so far as to say that modern civilization doesn't really have a culture at all, but merely a set of ideas and narratives that support profit-maximizing corporate behavior. In this respect, culture as we once knew it no longer exists.

"NORMAL" IS OVER

In any case, the gig is up. The fossil-fueled, profit-driven, culturally sanctioned house-wrecking party of the last 200 years is over. We are in crisis now and there's no place to hide. Our lives will never be the same again. There will be no going back to "normal" and in fact, as we stand at the edge of the abyss, many of us have come to the realization that "normal" was actually the driver of our predicament in the first place.

At this point, there is no easy fix and there's probably not even be a hard fix. As climate activist Rupert Read has put it, "Ashes are now inevitable." We can try to unknow or ignore this reality, but this predicament isn't going anywhere. No superhero or technological Santa Claus is going to come and rescue us. In short, the planet we grew up on no longer exists. As one quipster put it, "Carl Sagan's pale blue dot is about to become a hot red dot."

This encounter with The Knowledge radically revises—or should revise—our everyday psychology and our interactions with one another. In "normal," pre-crisis conditions, we were quick to comfort our children, our friends, and even strangers in distress with the soothing encouragement "It's all going to be OK." But in this case, it's not going to be OK; not even close to OK. In other words, this circumstance calls for a radical revision in the way we see the world, ourselves, and our ways of living. We need to turn our minds around, accept reality as it is, and yet, keep showing up with our best efforts. It's a big ask, but we really have no other choice. Radical change is coming, soon.

EPIC FAIL

These rude awakenings, inconvenient and disturbing as they are, are widely available to anyone who cares to look. Anyone who's even slightly curious about the state of the planet and their personal future should be able to learn the fundamentals without much effort. And yet, many of us fail to grasp the depth, magnitude, urgency, and gravity of our predicament. Many people fail to experience The Encounter at all, while others simply look away, unmoved.

Perhaps it's no wonder. Modern human attention has become radically fragmented and wickedly unstable. What's left of our native intelligence now leaps chaotically, always chasing the latest digital novelty, jumping from one distraction to the next, frantically trying to keep pace with the flashing lights, alerts and demands on our time. Chained to our devices, we're divorced from here and now realities. As MIT professor Sherry Turkle puts it in *Reclaiming Conversation*, "we are forever elsewhere."

And of course, many of us are living in our own informational and social silos, facilitated by our shiny devices. With a few swipes and taps, we program our phones to tell us precisely what we want to hear. It's a perfect circle of convenience and comfort; our devices reinforce our beliefs and keep us protected from any contradiction that might disturb our equanimity—no inconvenient truths or nasty encounters with The Knowledge to upset us. Life is good.

To make matters worse, corporate media is mostly missing in action on the biggest story in human history. Given the urgency, magnitude and stakes involved, we might expect to see headlines in every media outlet, every day. We'd expect to see writers, pundits and politicians talking about the atmosphere and the biosphere with every breath and keystroke, and very little else.

But the state of the planet is presented—if it's presented at all—as just another issue, equivalent in significance to all other issues. In this view, all stories are essentially equal, no matter their gravity or consequences. Urgent scientific warnings about a collapsing biosphere are not considered particularly newsworthy, especially when there's a celebrity drama in the works. Radical warming, extreme weather, sea level rise, desertification, the collapse of fisheries and agriculture—all of it gets pigeon-holed under "science stories" and pushed to the back of the queue.

Even worse, entertainment media has hijacked our brains and our culture. As a people, we're floundering, adrift in a world of superficial appearances, glitter, gloss, and shallow pleasure. Trivia, drama, and celebrity now take priority over substance, a trend famously described by media critic Neil Postman in his landmark 1985 book *Amusing Ourselves to Death*. As Postman saw it, modern society is sliding ever deeper into an entertainment-centric sinkhole in which rational discourse and deep experience are abandoned in favor of spectacle, gossip, and shlock; our intellectual discourse now reduced to bumper sticker slogans, hats and T-shirts.

So perhaps it's no great surprise to see widespread apathy and disengagement in the face of looming and accelerating catastrophe. Most people seem unmoved by scientific reports, data, exponential curves, and warnings from the world's top experts. We seem immune to reality and incredibly, a great many people don't even believe that a problem exists. As biologist and author George Tsakraklides has put it, "Humanity is not simply in denial. It has stopped paying attention altogether."

Even worse, there even seems to be an unspoken taboo against speaking about the biosphere at all. Or to put it another way, the natural world now lies outside our Overton window of acceptable discourse. It's almost unheard of for a politician or other prominent leader to talk about biology, natural life-supporting systems, ecology, biodiversity, carrying capacity, habitat, or human relations with the living world. Perhaps some have attempted it, only to be shouted down and marginalized by human supremacists and economic imperialists. Judging from the speech of our leaders and influencers, we might even suppose that the natural world doesn't actually exist, or if it does exist, it's nothing to worry about. This is what Adam McKay, producer of the film *Don't Look Up*, has called "the sonic boom of silence."

WHAT DID YOU DO?

The tragic fact is that many, if not most, people in the modern world are fundamentally uninformed or mis-informed about the most consequential event in human history. Nevertheless, humans do have some measure of free will, which is to say, in the age of highly accessible information, ignorance is not simply an accidental, incidental by-product of our fast-paced lifestyle—it's a choice. For those who want to know the state of the world, The Knowledge is there for the taking. All we have to do is pay attention.

Ultimately, our encounter with The Knowledge changes us. Or it doesn't. The understanding transforms us. Or it doesn't. We can accept the challenge and respond accordingly, or we can lapse back into the comfort, familiarity, convenience, and amusement of the modern world. It's up to us.

For some, The Knowledge can become a dreadful weight that drags us down and makes us miserable. But for others, it inspires a form of sacred, functional rage that integrates the entire mind-body-spirit. An asset and an ally, it can clarify, motivate and give us focus in the midst of ambiguity and extremity. It can help us triage, set priorities and avoid distraction. It can even make us whole.

In any case, humanity is faced with a stark choice: we can live as if reality matters, or we can protect, dodge, and weave. We can hide out in distraction and denial, fueled by hopium, or we can live a life of relevance. The poet Drew Dellinger throws down the gauntlet and makes the challenge crystal clear with a koan for our age: "What did you do once you knew?"

PATHS

You are what you risk.

Michele Wucker

So you've had your encounter with The Knowledge, but now what? What are you going to do with this radically inconvenient realization, this punishing series of rude awakenings? How will you respond to the greatest challenge in human history, this existential threat to the biosphere and life as we know it?

There are myriad possibilities and we all try to adapt in our own way. For some, the encounter is overwhelming and sets off an instant reaction of self-protection, alienation, denial, depression, and withdrawal. The weight of the world is just too much to bear, too inconvenient to accept, too intimidating to live with. For others, the experience will stimulate action, creativity and a heightened sense of responsibility. Still others will struggle and squirm, trying desperately to find some clarity, relevance, and meaning. Nevertheless, there are three common paths or archetypes that concern us here: the inactivist, the warrior, and the artivist. Understanding these responses will help us find a way forward.

THE INACTIVIST

Doing nothing risks everything.
Extinction Rebellion

Sentiment without action is the ruin of the soul.
Edward Abbey

Inactivism is by far the weakest path, but also the most popular—so popular in fact, that many of us will be slow to recognize it as anything unusual, deviant or abnormal. It's the default position for many, and as such, tends to be invisible. Nevertheless, it's essential that we recognize this response for its character and especially, its consequences.

On contact with The Knowledge, the inactivist mostly just shrugs. Disengaged, unmoved and inert, he lives on the sidelines of life and tries to keep his head down. Strangely indifferent to suffering and conditions outside his immediate orbit, he's passive in the face of unfolding catastrophe and is perfectly willing to let the planet go down without a fight.

When confronted by big, worldly challenges, the inactivist protests "It's not my job." Let others take care of the Earth, society and culture. Let the market fix it. Let government or the non-profits fix it. Let talk radio, Silicon Valley, or Hollywood fix it. And above all, let future generations fix it.

In essence, the inactivist sleepwalks through life, incurious about the monstrous systemic threats that lie just outside his door. He's not really interested in the history, origins, or back stories of how things got to be this way. He asks no questions, conducts no inquiry. Life is mostly just a spectator sport and he's nothing more than an innocent bystander.

When faced with inconvenient truths about the state of the planet, or anything else for that matter, the inactivist deploys a robust set of psycho-spiritual defense mechanisms that keep unpleasant realities at bay. Selective attention is his favorite method. The glass is half full, he reminds himself; keep your eye on the good things in life and don't get distracted by complex problems. Declare your innocence and above all, keep an upbeat, positive attitude. In the process, the inactivist greenwashes himself and by contagion, those around him.

For the dedicated inactivist, denial—either hard or soft—is the tool of choice. Either deny the science outright, or just let it slide. Things can't possibly be as bad as the scientists tell us. If things really were so bad, someone would have done something by now. And besides, it can't be real because, well, think how inconvenient that would be. Likewise, inactivists are largely addicted to hopium in all its various forms. "There are brilliant people out there working on the problem of clean energy" they tell us. "Green growth is the solution." Innovation is the cure for all that ails us; technology will save us.

All of which contributes to a state of willful or semi-willful ecological blindness. When confronted by inconvenient truths, it's easier to simply avoid the whole thing. Why go in search of information that's disturbing? Why seek out scientific reports that challenge our culture and our individual lifestyles? Why look into ideas that call into question capitalism, consumerism, fossil fuels, and the assumptions of human supremacy? Life is just a whole lot easier if we look on the bright side. Just pick the right cherries, the comforting stories, the easy opinions, the convenient products, and carry on.

At a basic level, the inactivist is passive, conflict avoidant, and domesticated—an ideal consumer. He chooses comfort over engagement, even if it means living in a state of irrelevance. No matter whether it's personal relationships or large-scale politics, he avoids anything that might provoke a push-back. He prefers to wait, in Martin Luther King Jr.'s words, for a "more convenient season." Perhaps engagement will be easier and more palatable at some later date.

In any case, comfort and security are his top priorities. To be active is to differ, but difference implies risk and is therefore unacceptable—an orientation sometimes described as *safetyism*. In *The Coddling of the American Mind*, authors Greg Lukianoff and Jonathan Haidt defined safetyism as a culture or belief system in which safety is held as a sacred value; risk is simply out of the question. No matter the domain or challenge, the inactivist avoids anything that might prove difficult or unpleasant.

In essence, inactivism is a retreat from reality. It's a retreat to business-as-usual, culture-as-usual, life-as-usual, and comfort-as-usual. When confronted by challenge and ambiguity, the inactivist returns to familiar, known conditions, even if those conditions are fundamentally dangerous or unhealthy. As he might well put it, "Better the devil you know than the one you don't."

Likewise, the inactivist is quick to a retreat to familiar narratives, especially comforting man-over-nature stories of human exceptionalism and technological salvation.

And when the going gets tough, he's quick to seek refuge in the plastic, consumeristic narratives that drive so much of our modern lives. When afflicted by doubt or anxiety, just buy something.

Likewise, the inactivist retreats into the self by focusing the lion's share of his effort on his individual welfare. The world is just too complicated to deal with, so he concentrates his attention on the hyper-local: his body, his personal life, his fitness, and his finances. In the process, he feathers his own nest, polishes his own apple and lives, as the magazines tell us, his "best life." In the extreme, this retreat from the larger world becomes a form of narcissism and in turn, an anti-solution. When millions of people retreat into their personal lives, community-based, systemic solutions become impossible.

A SHALLOW LIFE

Obviously, inactivism is a common orientation and behavior, but how do we understand it? What's the origin story—the etiology—of this affliction? Is it a simple lifestyle choice, a personality disorder or a character flaw? Is it a mental illness or a psycho-spiritual disorder? Is it cowardice? Is it normal?

As we've seen, active engagement is proof of life as well as evidence of wildness, vitality, and even sanity itself. But when activism is absent, we begin to wonder... Is this animal behaving normally? Wouldn't a healthy human animal push back against an assault on its life support systems? Is it accurate to call inactivism a psycho-spiritual disease? An epidemic? Should it be listed in the DSM, the *Diagnostic and Statistical Manual of Mental Disorders*, the bible of the therapy world? Maybe so.

But no matter what pigeonhole we put it in, there are big consequences and a terrible price to be paid, both collectively and personally. Most obviously, inactivism draws us down into a sinkhole of moral irrelevance. The inactivist thinks that his silence makes him safe, but it's actually a spiritual disaster that will degrade his sense of meaning and even his health. Even worse, it lends power to perpetrators of social and ecological trauma.

This is familiar ground in the world of civil rights and spirituality, as noted by some of our most prominent elders:

Martin Luther King, Jr.: "Our lives begin to end the day we become silent about things that matter." Likewise, "The way of acquiescence leads to moral and spiritual suicide."

Simone de Beauvoir: "The oppressor would not be so strong if he did not have accomplices among the oppressed."

Hannah Arendt: "Evil thrives on apathy and cannot exist without it."

Eleanor Roosevelt: "When you cease to make a contribution, you begin to die."

Desmond Tutu: "If you are neutral in situations of injustice, you have chosen the side of the oppressor."

Albert Einstein: "If I were to remain silent, I'd be guilty of complicity."

Elie Wiesel: "Always take sides. Neutrality helps the oppressor, never the victim. Silence encourages the tormentor, never the tormented."

NASA scientist and climate activist Peter Kalmus: "If you're 'neutral' at this point, you're complicit."

Naturally, critics will push back against the suggestion that ecological destruction is equivalent to civil rights abuses, tyranny or racism, but the comparison is perfectly apt. Destroying the habitability of the planet in no less evil than any other injustice or violence that humans perpetrate on one another. To kill a life-support system is to kill the people who depend upon it. In other words, ecocide *is* genocide.

Even worse, the inactivist's silence is infectious and feeds on itself in a spiral of disengagement and avoidance. Humans are herd animals; people don't talk about our ecological crisis precisely because people aren't talking about our ecological crisis.

The inactivist believes that neutrality and independence are both possible and desirable, but this is a fundamental misunderstanding of how the world works. As hyper-social animals, everything humans do is contagious. Like it or not, everything we do is political and influential in one way or another.

To put it another way, *activism is inevitable.* Everything we do touches the world in some manner; we are always creating and influencing the people around us. Slackers think they're being neutral, but they're really perpetuating the status quo. Inactivists believe they're safe, but in their passivity, they're voting for a path to a radically dysfunctional, catastrophic future.

Ultimately, inactivism becomes a path to moral irrelevance and even ill-health. It's often said that "activism is the antidote to despair" but it's also true that inactivism is a formula for depression and a life of meaninglessness. It's not just a failure to contribute, it's also a personal catastrophe and a slippery slope to spiritual ruin.

Even worse perhaps, the inactivist fails to discover who he really is. Without engagement, there can be no self-discovery or self-awareness. Without risk and participation, the inactivist will never come to understand his true capabilities, aptitudes, or inclinations. This is the origin of his identity crisis and ultimately, his suffering.

On one level, the inactivist response to planetary disaster is perfectly understandable. Modern humans are already highly distracted, chronically stressed, and struggling to make a go of it in wickedly abnormal, alien environment. Many of us are effectively paralyzed by cognitive overload, anxiety, and trauma, so it's no surprise that millions of people are deploying their defense mechanisms, feasting on hopium and reverting to the familiar. In this condition, taking on another psychic and spiritual challenge, especially one of such immense proportions, might well be unbearable.

But just because a thing is explainable or understandable doesn't make it right. Just because a thing is commonplace doesn't make it healthy. We can and must do better. So beware—if you choose the path of inactivism, you're not just ghosting the planet and future generations, you're also ghosting yourself, your body, and your loved ones. It's not a good way to live.

THE WAY OF THE WARRIOR

We are born into a dangerous time. You can
consider it an affliction or an assignment.

Stephen Jenkinson

As we've seen, the inactivist responds to his encounter
with The Knowledge by withdrawing, isolating, and denying reality. It's a shallow way of life, one that leads to
despair and ultimately, irrelevance. In contrast, today's
ecological warrior is fully alive and awake to the depth,
magnitude and urgency of our predicament. Driven by a
compelling sense of urgency, she's assertive and focused in
her orientation and her actions; she shows up with every
cell in her body. The Knowledge is a constant presence in
her life, a reminder that clarifies, focuses and motivates.

The eco-warrior may be new on the scene, but she's actually part of a long and noble tradition that stretches back
many thousands of years. Warriors have always stood up
for their people and the land they inhabit. Today's challenge may be more complex and global in scope, but the
primary mission remains the same. In this, the modern
eco-warrior becomes a protector and a defender, not just
of a local region, but of the entire biosphere, the land, air,
and water of her tribe, the people of the Earth.

Living in that tradition and spirit, today's Earth warrior
is resolute and determined, radically sincere and committed to action. She's not just risk tolerant, but actually embraces the challenge and ambiguity that goes with engagement. She understands the dangers clearly; she may be
shunned, arrested, exiled or punished with financial ruin.

She may be misunderstood, unappreciated, and she may well fail in her efforts. Nevertheless, she persists.

The warrior identifies with striving and struggle and in a sense, lives to fight. Her revolutionary spirit runs white hot, and she stands ready and willing to challenge power at every opportunity. She speaks out and speaks up, refusing to be pinned down by convention, habit, conditioning, or domestication. Her resolve is central to her identity and she refuses to go gently into that good—or not so good—night.

Ultimately, the warrior understands that participation is the secret to life and that safetyism is nothing more than a seductive fantasy. In this perspective, she stands with Helen Keller:

> Security is mostly a superstition. It does not exist in nature, nor do the children of men as a whole experience it. Avoiding danger is no safer in the long run than outright exposure. Life is either a daring adventure, or nothing.

THE SHADOW SIDE

The warrior's willingness to sacrifice personal welfare for the health of her people and the planet is honorable and possibly even health-promoting. Along the way, she not only serves her people and future generations, she also discovers what she's made of. In the process of engagement, she learns a great deal about her identity, her capabilities, inclinations, and weaknesses. In a very real sense, she discovers who she is.

It's a noble path, but there's danger in the warrior's orientation, especially in the way that her passion can drive her body, her thinking and her actions. Her intensity is essential, but it can also be alienating, not just to adversaries, but even to allies. Even worse, her commitment can harden into dogma, fundamentalism, rigidity and hyper-vigilance. When the cause becomes everything, the warrior's demeanor can become increasingly humorless, even grim. Consumed by the urgency of the moment, her character can even morph into grandiosity and narcissism.

The warrior's dedication also puts her at risk of falling into a confrontational mind and spirit set. Laser-focused on perpetrators and objectives, she begins to think of the world exclusively as a zero-sum game; it's always win-lose, us-versus-them. In turn, this can make for some bad martial artistry as her adversarial orientation hardens into tunnel vision and binary, black and white thinking. This can lead to a contraction of the imagination, precisely at a time when we need it most.

Likewise, the warrior mindset inclines us towards militant thinking and militarized language. As the climate crisis intensifies, more and more people are calling for a "WWII style mobilization" and the need to be on a "war footing." And while the need for some kind of massive mobilization is clear, this kind of language is surely counterproductive. Have we forgotten the brutality of war and the suffering that goes with it? Isn't there a more creative metaphor we can promote?

For the warrior, the intensive focus on destinations and objectives is laudable and sometimes effective, but it can also devolve into ends-over-means thinking. The end— some kind of functional future for the planet—is so vital that it would seem to justify almost any kind of action.

But cutting corners and bending our values for the sake of victory can have unintended, catastrophic side effects. We may prevail over adversaries in the moment, but if our path and process is ugly, this too will have consequences.

In her intensity, the warrior brings powerful focus to the perpetrators of our age, as she must; their behaviors must be contained, and the sooner the better. But a vital question looms: What comes after success? If all we do is tear down existing systems, we're left with a power vacuum that my well devolve into something even more destructive than the original affliction. In her passion and enthusiasm for change, the warrior might inadvertently open the gates for something even more horrific.

In the process, the warrior can even lose sight of the original goal—protecting that which she loves and values. The English writer G. K. Chesterton put it best: "A true warrior fights not because he hates what is in front of him, but because he loves what is behind him." In our fervor to prevail against our adversaries, we risk forgetting the things that we value, the things that led us to engagement in the first place. It's a kind of amnesia: When we become obsessed with the corporate-ecocidal-big-power adversaries in front of us, we run the risk of losing our biophilia, our intense love for the living earth and the people who live here.

Not only that, the warrior's constant striving can even degrade her psycho-physical health. With relentless effort, the human nervous system never gets a chance to metabolize experience and rebuild itself. This is something every athletic coach knows full well: periods of intense striving must alternate with periods of deep rest. In other words, the process must be rhythmic.

Likewise, the warrior orientation tends to generate intense stress, both within the body and in relationships. When conflicts are frequent and the stakes are high, the warrior's intensity can even lead to an affliction sometimes described as the "John Henry syndrome." As the story goes, John Henry was a legendary railroad worker who went head-to-head against a steam-powered drilling machine and in the process literally worked himself to death. The syndrome has been described by public health researchers as "a strategy for coping with prolonged exposure to stresses by expending high levels of effort which results in accumulating physiological costs."

For the warrior, the stress of full-time, full-contact activism can be exhilarating, seductive, and manageable for a time, but the chronic striving will eventually lead to burn out, exhaustion, and eventually, depression. In turn, she becomes vulnerable to a condition psychologists recognize as "learned helplessness." When the human animal suffers a long string of defeats in which escape is impossible, it eventually comes to assume failure, even in easily manageable situations. This is a catastrophe for the body and the spirit, as well as the spirits of those around us.

In the extreme, frequent failure can also lead to cynicism and the dead-end belief that nothing really matters. On bad days, we come to believe that the problem of our age is humanity, full stop. Humans are smart enough to invent powerful tools, but too stupid to use them wisely. People are motivated purely by self-interest and greed. And on it goes, circling into yet another quagmire of misanthropy and bitterness. At this point, there's no energy or creativity left to work with and not much point in carrying on. No future is possible, so what's the point in trying?

All that's left is to call it a day and retreat into distraction, sloth and inactivism.

The warrior's path is righteous and we are right to honor this fighting spirit and dedication to the cause—the Earth, the biosphere, and a functional future. If even a few more people showed the courage of the activist warrior, the outlook for our future would look a lot less bleak. Nevertheless, it's also true that the warrior orientation can become a health-negative that leads us into a psycho-spiritual black hole. The warrior's sacrifice is noble, but when taken to an extreme, it also diminishes and dilutes our power. When we give everything to the cause and burn with too much intensity, we aren't going to be much use to anyone, much less the planet as a whole.

In other words, the warrior's way—when taken to an extreme—may not be sustainable. After all, it's hard to have a healthy, full life when you're constantly on a war footing. Perhaps a more well-rounded approach would serve us better...

THE WAY OF THE ARTIVIST

The artivist uses her artistic talents to fight and struggle against injustice and oppression—by any medium necessary. The artivist merges commitment to freedom and justice with the pen, the lens, the brush, the voice, the body, and the imagination. The artivist knows that to make an observation is to have an obligation.

M. K. Asante

If I can't dance at your revolution, I'm not coming.

Emma Goldman

As we've seen, the warrior spirit is honorable and for some, an ideal path to relevance and effective action. But the orientation is not for everyone and might not even serve us well in the long run. High-intensity engagement is vital, but there also needs to be a sense of balance and proportion to keep us whole. So perhaps there's another way to live in this world, a way that's effective, creative, meaningful, health-promoting, and sustainable. With this in mind, imagine a creative activist or *artivist*, someone who's ready to step up and put their imagination to work in the fight for a functional future and a meaningful life.

In fact, at this point in history, a creative orientation is absolutely essential. Today's challenges aren't just unique in recent human history, they're unique in the totality of the human experience. Never before have we faced this particular combination of physics, biology, society and culture. Everything is in flux now and conventional rules of behavior no longer apply. As author Naomi Klein has put it "No is not enough." Resistance is necessary and honorable but is not sufficient. Today the call to humanity might well be described as a simple binary: *create or die*.

Unfortunately, the words *art* and *creativity* come with some heavy and highly distracting baggage. People think of art as nothing more than pretty pictures and even worse, believe that it's only for special people who are somehow "gifted" or "creative." But these assumptions sabotage our efforts at the root. Not only do they limit what we create, they also hamstring our ability to move society and culture. In fact, art and creativity are intrinsic to the human experience and are absolutely essential in our fight for a functional future.

IMAGINATION IN ACTION

Like the warrior, the artivist is awake to the urgency and gravity of our predicament and embraces responsibility that goes with it. His revolutionary spirit burns bright, but is expressed in original ways. Like the warrior, he understands that participation is the secret to life, but the fight is just the beginning. He's focused on perpetrators and the alpha problems of our age, but he's also intrigued by large-scale systems, consciousness and culture. Never seduced by the front stories of commercial culture, he's deeply curious and is always asking questions. He reads and studies the history, back stories and origin stories of how we got here. He wants to know the big picture.

For the artivist, The Knowledge remains a demanding challenge, but it's also a form of raw material for his work. Every crisis, every intractable problem, every systemic breakdown, every failure of culture-as-usual; these are starting points and inspirations for his work. Dedicated to acts of creative subversion and rebellion, the artivist is resilient and forward thinking. He's just as intimidated by the state of the planet as anyone else but finds power and meaning in the artistic endeavor.

For the artivist, the beauty of engagement is that it's a wide open opportunity for creative expression. There's no textbook here, no academic degree, no authorities, no recipe for best practices. In other words, it's not a hard science. No one can tell us how to do activism with any kind of precision; there's simply too many unknowns and too much dynamism in the systems we're working with. But far from being an obstacle, this makes it an ideal domain for art and creativity. In this sense, the modern world is a blank canvas for our creative efforts.

In a world of hard ball politics, this creative orientation might seem soft, artsy, and ineffective, but it's actually a powerful method for dealing with the monumental challenges of our age. For the artivist, creative action stems from an understanding of complex systems in the social and natural world. As we've seen, these systems often behave in non-linear ways. Strict cause-and-effect descriptions are inadequate to describe how these systems actually behave; butterfly effects are always in play, sometimes generating surprising outcomes. In this way, every work of art, whether physical, graphic, musical, or performative has the potential to become larger than itself. When art works, it moves people in ways that rational language and action cannot.

Like the warrior, the artist maintains a focus on ends and objectives, but means are just as important and by some calculations, maybe even more so. In other words, beauty, pleasure, dignity, and wisdom in the process are vital. Even in defeat, the quality of our creativity can endure and cascade outward. In the long run, a beautiful defeat might be even more influential and persuasive than an ugly victory.

The artivist understands the gravity of our predicament and the need for swift, effective action, but manages to maintain a playful spirit in strategy, tactics, relationships and action. He's dead serious about the urgency of our situation, but he also understands the value of creative humor, laughter, and celebratory, life-affirming experience.

To the average ear, this light-hearted, playful approach might sound trivial and completely inappropriate for meeting the epic, life-threatening demands of our age, but there's nothing to say that we can't be dead serious, resolute and playful at the same time. In fact, this might well be exactly the spirit we're looking for.

The beauty of the playful approach is that it helps us maintain our balance and equanimity, even in the face of titanic adversity. It also helps us to transcend false endpoints—assumptions that limit our imagination and in turn, our effectiveness. Even better, a playful orientation communicates a sense of safety to the people around us, both allies and adversaries.

As a lateral thinker, the artivist is less likely to get locked into the binary trap of forward-backward, advance-retreat that can bedevil the warrior. In the world of traditional martial arts, this is called "getting off the line." The artist's body is threatened by a kick or a punch, so he shifts his position to the left or right without giving up his integrity. He's not fleeing and he's not attacking; merely repositioning himself to create new possibilities and opportunities for movement.

Likewise, the artivist thinks in terms of creative work-arounds. A direct engagement might waste his time and energy, so why not create something completely novel? This was the approach advocated by Buckminster Fuller, creator of tensegrity structures such as the geodesic dome. As he saw it, "You never change things by fighting the existing reality. To change something, build a new model that makes the existing model obsolete." In other words, the artivist creates *around* his adversary.

All of which gives us a fresh, maybe even liberating perspective. With a creative workaround, you can almost ignore your adversary, at least for a time; you've got more important things to do. And in this effort, the artivist might even come to see his opponents as less problematic and frightening. To be sure, adversaries still matter and it's wise to keep an eye on their movements, but they might turn out to be less of a threat than first imagined.

Naturally, process is vital and this is where the artivist practices the art of *bricolage*, using whatever's available to advance his creation. In this practice, he doesn't worry about styles, standard methods, best practices, or convention. Rather, he opens his mind to possibility, innovation, and outrageous combinations. He doesn't get distracted or tyrannized by optimal techniques but works with whatever he's got on hand: allies, resources, ideas, materials or information. Even more importantly, he doesn't much care that he doesn't have the right skills, the right materials, or the right training. He seizes the opportunities that come his way and tries his best.

Not surprisingly, the artivist is also deeply suspicious of rigid taxonomies and the general boxification of nearly everything in the modern world. Pigeonholes are all well and good, but they also limit what we can see and do. Once we're in a box, our thinking and creative vagility is compromised. We've been captured, incarcerated, hog-tied, maybe even domesticated. And once we've been rigidly defined, labeled, and categorized, our creativity is dead. This is the tyranny of genre.

The conventional, inside-the-box solution is to "think outside the box," but the artivist goes further and is skeptical of *all* pigeonholes, boilerplate language, templates, disciplinary boundaries, and ready-made forms that will further boxify and constrain his efforts. As Bruce Lee famously described his martial philosophy, "One can function freely and totally only if he is 'beyond system.' The man who is really serious, with the urge to find out what truth is, has no style at all. He lives only in what is."

UPSIDES

The artistic path can be extremely powerful, both at the inner and outer levels of our experience, and it's almost certainly less stressful than that of the warrior. The artivist is still vulnerable to defeat, despair and depression as we all are, but the effect is buffered by the possibilities for creative novelty and engagement of the imagination. This adds up to less stress and better health in the long run.

For the artivist, there's simply more room in his thinking and his experience. He's less likely to get trapped in adversarial binaries or zero-sum approaches to life. This translates into a greater ease, resilience, and the ability to endure the inevitable hardships that come with engagement. As the artivist might put it, "Whatever doesn't kill me makes me more creative."

The playful spirit can also give us a greater sense of control and agency in the face of overwhelming odds. As we've seen, the modern activist is fighting an uphill battle against vastly more powerful forces; defeats are common and may even lead us into a state of learned helplessness. But when the creative spirit is alive, options give us room to breathe and maybe even feed on themselves with an increased sense of possibility.

INTEGRATION

I have found purpose in a world that often seems empty and meaningless to so many people.

Greta Thunberg

The most important days of your life: The day you are born and the day you find out why.

Mark Twain

As we've seen, the path of inactivism leads to a shallow life that only serves to deepen our sense of irrelevance and despair. On the other hand, the way of the warrior can harden into zealotry, dogma, rigidity, exhaustion, and burn out. Artivism sounds like an ideal solution, but even this path carries immense challenges.

So the question before us: How do we turn our activism into a relevant, health-positive experience that's both effective and good for our bodies? Should activism be included as a part of modern medical practice? Should physicians write prescriptions for active engagement with the world? How does activism fit with other more familiar health practices? And most importantly, can activism make us whole?

At this point, it helps to step back and take a closer look at ideas of holistic health that have come and gone over the ages, beginning with native and indigenous people. In traditional cultures, the model is expansive and emphasizes continuity with the world: mind, body, spirit, land, tribe and ancestry are held to be essential elements of this holistic view. Native people assume a permeability and dialogue between inside and outside, internal and external. In this perspective, the skin is not a boundary or a barrier, but a sensing organ, a living link to the natural world. In fact, the work of the traditional shaman was radically inclusive: the objective was nothing less than to realign the body with the flux and flow of the cosmos.

This integrated view held sway for millennia but was largely eclipsed with the rise of scientific medicine. Spectacular discoveries in microbiology vanquished some of our most dread diseases and set the stage for a new age of biomedicine. Almost overnight, our attention narrowed to the domains of biochemistry, physiology, genetics and technological innovation. Much was gained in the process, but many people began to suspect that something vital was being lost. Health improved for millions, but many of us no longer felt whole.

Today we see a renewed interest in integration and a wide variety of holistic formulations, all of them aimed at recovering our lost sense of unity. In 1977, pioneering physician George Engel advanced a *biopsychosocial* model as an alternative to the prevailing biomedical approach. Engel recognized the power of context, setting, and predicament on the human organism and encouraged the modern physician to take a more expansive view of medical practice.

Likewise, we've all heard the popular mind-body-spirit model for holistic health. This formulation is more expansive than the biomedical model—a step in the right direction—but it fails to include the world outside the body, especially our life supporting systems of habitat, atmosphere, and biosphere. Even worse, the model has largely been co-opted by powerful corporate interests whose primary objective is to sell products and services. In this respect, the commercialized mind-body-spirit formula isn't really about health at all. In fact, it mostly serves to contract our awareness and sabotage our efforts at genuine integration.

In our highly individualistic, Big Me culture, health and integration are considered to be mostly, if not exclusively, personal concerns. It's *my* body, *my* mind, *my* spirit. Integration is something that happens inside me; if I can get my mind, body, and spirit working together, I'll be whole. But this view utterly fails to capture the totality of the human animal, living in context. In essence, it's a form of isolation. For us to be whole, there has to be a recognition and appreciation for the outside circles that sustain our lives: tribe, habitat, and the natural world in particular.

Fortunately, other models give us more guidance. For example, the "One Health" model is an interdisciplinary alliance of progressive veterinarians, physicians and other health professionals. This collaboration emphasizes the shared welfare of humans, non-human animals, and their habitat. It also argues for multi-disciplinary approaches to prevention, education, and policy development. Much of the work in One Health has focused on infectious diseases and the spread of pathogens, but it's safe to assume continuities across the animal kingdom. If you improve the health of habitat, you improve the health of all the animals—including humans—within that habitat.

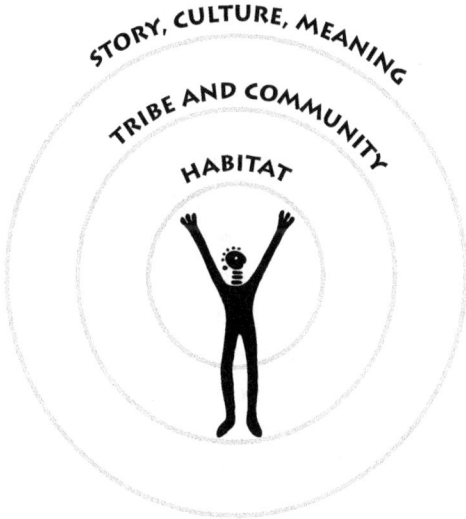

STORY, CULTURE, MEANING
TRIBE AND COMMUNITY
HABITAT

Then there's the concentric model of holism, based on three life-supporting rings that surround the human body. The inner-most ring is habitat, including atmosphere and biosphere. Obviously, this is essential to human function and it scarcely needs to be said that without a functioning habitat, there can be no health, no economy, or any other human endeavor for that matter.

The second ring of life-support includes our people, our tribes and our communities. This is also essential; as hyper-social animals, social contact is vital for maintaining our sense of belonging and our mental health.

The third ring consists of story, narrative and our sense of meaning, embedded in culture and our life experience. This is also a true life-supporting system; without a unifying narrative and sense of purpose, we tend to drift aimlessly and our bodies become weak. This model, so simple in its design, cuts through much of our confusion, giving us essential guidance and a sense of coherence.

HEALTH IS INDIVISIBLE

These holistic models vary in the details, but they all point towards a comprehensive, integrative approach. Intuitively, we know that our health must be well-rounded; if we put too much emphasis on any one element, the effort becomes unbalanced. But the curious thing about these models is that none of them explicitly include engagement with the world. Where is the activism? Aren't we missing something vital? How did we come to overlook something so crucial in the health and functioning of the human animal, especially when there's a solid body of work connecting our sense of meaning and purpose with good health outcomes? This is quite possibly the biggest oversight in the world of modern health and medicine.

It will take some time to re-write and re-imagine our models of holistic health, but in the meantime, maybe the best approach is to follow the lead of writer and environmental activist Wendell Berry. As he saw it, "Health is indivisible." In other words, everything in our world has a role to play in the functioning of our lives. That is, all parts of the human experience—both inside and outside—are inter-related and interdependent. Everything we touch, eat, feel, say, hear, or do has the potential to influence how our bodies work or don't work. For Berry, human health included natural elements such as soil, water, and the myriad activities of plants and animals involved in farming, but we can be sure that Berry would have endorsed activism as a vital part of the circle. By taking on the challenges of our world, we knit the circle together into a single, unified whole. Participation is the glue that binds it all together.

INTEGRATE THE KLUDGE

To really understand the depth and importance of the holistic orientation, we'd do well to step back and learn a new word: kludge (or as it's sometimes spelled, kluge). Taken from the world of engineering and computer science, a kludge is a patched-together workaround or quick-and-dirty solution, often dismissed as clumsy, inelegant, inefficient, and hard to maintain. And while engineers are quick to heap scorn on the kludge, it can actually be a functional, practical way to solve difficult problems.

Out in the real world, we see kludges all around us. For example, the modern city is a kludge, a patched-together assembly of buildings, roads, tunnels, and parks—some planned, others improvised—that work together in a clunky kind of way. A remodeled house is also a kludge; add a bedroom this year, maybe a rec room or guest quarters over the garage the year after. It may not be as elegant as something planned entirely from scratch, but it mostly works. And of course, almost every computer on the planet is a hodgepodge of applications, customizations, workarounds and hacks that look ugly to the expert, but still manage to get the job done.

But what does this have to do with health and the human body and the human life? Surely our bodies are more unified than a city, a remodeled house or God-forbid, a computer hard drive. Actually, the similarities are remarkable. Take a look at our deep history and evolutionary origins and suddenly, we're struck by some astonishing realizations. That is, the body turns out to be many things—many systems—working together to produce our lives, our health, and our behavior.

Take, for example, the mitochondria that live in every cell of the body. These tiny organelles are responsible for producing the energy that drives metabolism. We might assume that they're our own creations and that they belong to us, but in fact, they contain their own DNA which is to say, they are separate organisms with their own history, operating in a symbiotic relationship within the human body. In other words, the human animal is a collaboration, not a single entity. We are many things, trying to work together as one.

Other examples abound. The stress response system—the hypothalamus, pituitary, adrenal axis—is also a patchwork. The digestive system, immune system, sensory system; all are incredibly efficient kludges in their own right. Even the brain is a collection of discrete layers—brainstem, midbrain, and cortex—each with its own history and function, cobbled together to create an impressive if somewhat unreliable organ. In short, nothing in the body was designed from scratch. It's all the result of evolutionary change operating over vast expanses of time; pieces working together more or less as one.

All of which helps us understand the challenge before us and the role that activism might play. Simply put, the prime objective in health, medicine, therapy and related arts is—or should be—integration. Can activism help the human kludge come together in a single, functional unity?

The good news is that we already know how this process works, or doesn't work. We know for example that certain activities and experiences tend to fragment the human organism into a state of disconnection and disintegration. Artificial light is notoriously disruptive, especially when it's out of step with the natural waxing and waning of circadian rhythms. Trauma, whether it be personal, intergenerational, or cultural also has a disintegrating effect as it disrupts normal, health-promoting patterns of attachment and safety. Meaningless stress also erodes our integration. As we've all experienced, the modern world presents us with a tsunami of mixed messages and in turn, puts us into a state of autonomic confusion. Whipsawed between fight-flight and rest-digest, the body scarcely knows what to do with itself, all of which is exacerbated by noise, distraction, acceleration, and the asynchronous communication and incoherent narratives generated by our electronic devices.

But tragically, all of these forces are highly embedded features of the modern world and it's very much correct to describe our modern world as a *disintegrative environment*. Many of us are quick to praise the comforts of modernity, but it's the incoherent nature of modern living that's driving us to pieces. In this sense, the remarkable thing is not the widespread prevalence of mental and physical health disorders that we see—what's truly amazing is that so many of us manage to remain substantially healthy in the face of such acutely disintegrating forces, processes, and challenges.

The good news is that we also know a great deal about the integrating forces that contribute to wholeness. We've heard the list a thousand times: Vigorous physical movement (aka "exercise") is especially integrating because it calls on the body to bring all its resources together into a single, concentrated effort. The deeper and more sustained the engagement, the more powerful the integrating effect. Then there's the integrating effect of natural light, circadian rhythm and especially, sleep. Meditation helps us integrate as well; sustained attention to the breath brings a sense of unity to mind and body. Social support, love, touch, and oxytocin move us toward integration, as does coherent culture, integrating narratives, sense of purpose, and meaningful stress.

All of this is well known and understood. What's less widely appreciated is the integrating power of engagement. In the simplest terms, activism is similar to a good physical workout. Like running, swimming, climbing, or weightlifting, confronting the status quo calls upon the animal to rally its forces and resources into the single doing of an act.

Imagine that you're about to engage in a high-profile action that challenges you in a new way; maybe an act of civil disobedience, an edgy talk before a live audience or a conflicted meeting with a powerful person. All of these encounters are going to put you under stress, and if you're smart, well-prepared, and lucky, it's going to be an optimal level of stress, something we call *eustress*. Do this repeatedly over the course of months and years, and your body will improve its ability to integrate. Over time, integration becomes a skill.

At this point it's important to remember that the specific

form of activism might not matter much. It's not as if writing a particular kind of letter or confronting a particular policymaker will drive your mind-body-spirit together into a single, cohesive whole. What does matter is the quality of our experience and especially, our level of exposure. It's the very act of going outside our comfort zone that calls the body to integration. In other words, easy doesn't work. Comfortable doesn't work. This is precisely why the inactivist is likely to be in sub-optimal health; camped out in his familiar comfort zone, his body has no incentive to integrate. What he needs is engagement and risk. Risk is what works.

MEANING AND PURPOSE

> When you act on behalf of something greater than yourself, you begin to feel it acting through you with a power that is greater than your own.
>
> Joanna Macy

But there's a lot more to the process of integration than simply getting the exposure right. As most of us are coming to realize, having a sense of meaning and purpose in life—and acting on that purpose—has powerfully unifying effect on the entire organism. This is precisely what Viktor Frankl observed while incarcerated in a prisoner of war camp in World War II. As recounted in his classic work *Man's Search for Meaning*, Frankl saw suffering everywhere. Men were starving and freezing, there was pain and misery in every moment and some were literally worked to death. Some men buckled under the strain and perished early, but others managed to live and even find fleeting moments of satisfaction in companionship. Frankl wondered, "Why do some survive while others weaken and die?"

His conclusion was that the survivors possessed a certain sense of meaning that animated their lives and helped them endure. He often quoted philosopher Friedrich Nietzsche: "He who has a why to live can transcend almost any how." Or, as we might say today, "He who has a why to live can tolerate almost any stressor." Or even further, "He who has a why to live can maintain his integrity and equipoise even in the face of powerful opponents and looming ecological collapse."

This insight has a powerful appeal to those of us living in today's hyper-stressed environment and it even suggests that having a "why" might well be the single most important factor in our ability to manage the ferocious, chronic complexity of the modern world. Suddenly, all our obsessive focus on diet, exercise, and other details of health begins to seem rather trivial and maybe even irrelevant. After all, none of the prisoners in Nazi concentration camps had anything resembling an optimal diet or exercise program. And yet, some of them managed to live and later thrive. Frankl himself lived to the age of ninety-two, animated, we can be sure, by his own powerful sense of why.

In fact, a growing body of evidence confirms the power of purpose and meaning in human health. In 2017, New Scientist magazine summarized the findings:

> People with a greater sense of purpose live longer, sleep better and have better sex. Purpose cuts

the risk of stroke and depression. It helps people recover from addiction or manage their glucose levels if they are diabetic. If a pharmaceutical company could bottle such a treatment, it would make billions.

In Japan they call it *ikigai*, "a reason for being." In short, it's our reason for getting out of bed in the morning. It's the juice that sustains us in conflict and keeps us going when we're up against formidable adversaries and long odds. Multiple studies have shown that ikigai has measurable health benefits and that individuals who believe their lives are worth living live longer.

A 2019 study reported in The Journal of the American Medical Association is typical: *Association Between Life Purpose and Mortality Among US Adults Older Than 50 Years*. As the authors put it,

> A growing body of literature suggests that having a strong sense of purpose in life leads to improvements in both physical and mental health and enhances overall quality of life. There are interventions available to influence life purpose; thus, understanding the association of life purpose with mortality is critical.

Obviously, activism is one such "intervention."

All of which takes us into some new psycho-cultural territory. In conventional, popular culture, pleasure is the name of the game and is aggressively sold to us as the ultimate goal. We want to feel good and we're quick to go in search of anything that promises more intense pleasure. Food, sex, alcohol, fun and amusement; these are the things that drive us. But sooner or later, most of us grow up and come to discover that pleasure doesn't really sustain or nourish us for long. It's welcome and it's worth pursuing, but on its own, it fails to give us the satisfaction that we're after. There must be something more.

Steven Cole, a researcher at the University of California, Los Angeles, studied the contrast in detail, comparing two types of well-being: *hedonic*, that which comes from the pursuit of pleasure, and *eudaemonic*, that which comes from having a purpose beyond self-gratification. The results showed that people with higher measures of hedonic well-being had higher expression of inflammatory genes and lower expression of genes for disease-fighting anti-bodies, a pattern also seen in loneliness and stress. For people scoring highest on eudaemonia, it was the opposite. Cole suspects that a focus on purpose decreases the nervous system's reaction to danger. Similar studies indicate that people with higher eudaemonic well-being have lower levels of the stress hormone cortisol. "Things that you value can override things that you fear," said Cole. In other words, it's beginning to look like hedonism is not the true path to health, stress-resistance, and resilience. What we really need is a powerful sense of why.

TO OR FROM?

To put it another way, we might well ask a simple question, grounded in the physical experience of our bodies. "Are you running away from something, or towards something? From the body's point of view, this makes an immense difference. Running away implies fear, stress, aversion, and resistance, all of which have a particular neurobiological profile. We may well have good reason to run from the lions, tigers and bears in our lives, but to do so constantly has a corrosive effect, not just on the tissue of our bodies, but on our cognition and our spirit. When running away, we close the aperture of our attention and think mostly in terms of urgency, scarcity, and short-term survival. This is not a good formula for creativity or activism.

In contrast, running towards something meaningful and purposeful will have a completely different neurochemical and spiritual result. Dopamine and serotonin surge as we're motivated by curiosity, desire, maybe even love and passion. This is not only good for our health, it's ideal for creative action.

So here's the crucial distinction: Are you running away from climate catastrophe and the imminent destruction of a habitable planet? Or are you running *towards* a new/old paradigm of biocentric relationships with the natural world? Are you running *away* from dysfunctional social systems and corporate dominance of society or are you running towards a system based on mutual cooperation and human universals? Obviously, some degree of running away will always be part of the human experience in any age, but it's the running towards that pulls the body together and keeps us whole.

COHERENCE

Speaking of meaning, purpose, and integration, a closely related concept is coherence, pioneered by Israeli-American sociologist Aaron Antonovsky. As he saw it, the state of the human animal depends primarily on lived experience and our relationship with the world as a whole:

> We are coming to understand health not as the
> absence of disease, but rather as the process
> by which individuals maintain their sense of
> coherence (i.e. sense that life is comprehensible,
> manageable, and meaningful) and ability to
> function in the face of changes in themselves and
> their relationships with their environment.

This sounds incredibly powerful, even more so than the conventional mind-body-spirit triad. It speaks to the primal experience of the human animal, born into a world without explanation. Life take us by surprise and then what? If our experience makes some kind of sense, if reality feels consistent and reliable, everything else tends to fall into place and the body simply works better.

So what of our experience in the modern world? Is it coherent? Comprehensible? Manageable? Meaningful? For many of us, the answer to all these questions is a resounding no. Radical complexity, cognitive overload, dysfunctional social systems, and looming ecological collapse add up to a crippling loss of coherence. It's no wonder that our psycho-physical health is suffering; our experience is fragmented and it's easy to lose our way. We might even go so far as to describe this lack of coherence as a planetary epidemic.

The good news is that activism can give us some of the coherence we're looking for. Start by taking one issue and making it your own. Learn the history, the facts, the players, and the conventions; this will make your experience *comprehensible*. Triage your efforts and choose your battles carefully; this will make your experience *manageable*. Work with others to take on the most important issues you can find; this will make your experience *meaningful*.

Going further, this coherence model would make a perfect formula for anyone who works with the human animal, especially in the worlds of education, athletics, and medicine. Therapists, teachers, coaches, trainers, and health professionals at all levels might well question the experience of their students, clients, and patients. Is their experience coherent? Can your program or organization help make their lives more comprehensible, controllable, and meaningful? If so, you're on the right path. If not, you've got some work to do.

LIFE-CENTRIC WHYS

Living in a world that's so often incoherent, it's easy to lose focus and flounder, but the good news is that most of us already have an appreciation for the power of meaning and purpose. It's a human universal to be moved by the big ideas of family, community, country, justice, and the quest for a better future. Intuitively and by experience, we seem to understand that life just works better when we focus on something bigger than ourselves. Likewise, we begin to see that the self-focused why of modern culture is abnormal and historically deviant. A narcissistic sense of purpose can drive us for a time, but it ultimately turns ugly, dysfunctional, and irrelevant. Frankl would surely have recognized the poverty of this kind of thinking and would have been quick to predict the demise of any self-focused prisoners in his camp.

But what now? Our familiar "whys" of family, friends,

and country are all well and good, but what's going to activate and sustain us in the face of imminent ecological catastrophe? What's the meaning and purpose that will animate our efforts and move us towards integration, coherence, and effectiveness in an extreme predicament?

Superficially, we might say that our mission is to "Save the Earth," but somehow, this one lacks the power to really move us. It's just too big, too daunting, and too vague. A better approach might be to look for meaning and purpose in the circle of life itself. In this, we can derive a profound sense of energy from a life-centric, kin-centric, biocentric orientation. Just as family, friends, and country can sustain our motivation in times of hardship, so too can our awareness of interdependence and deep participation in the epic drama of life on Earth.

The essential thing to understand is that life on Earth is a singular force. The plants and animals around us appear to be diverse and separate individuals, but in fact, they're part of a unitary process of generation, a biological tsunami that has swept across the globe in a 3 billion year wave of outrageous creativity. Rachel Carson put it perfectly:

> To understand biology is to understand that all life
> is linked to the Earth from which it came; it is to
> understand that the stream of life, flowing out of
> the dim past into the uncertain future, is in reality
> a unified force, though composed of an infinite
> number and variety of separate lives.

If we could feel, or at least appreciate, the depth, power, and magnificence of biological life, we'd be energized and integrated at an entirely new level. When you've got the biosphere at your back, almost anything becomes possible. When life itself is your ally, there's no limit to what you can do.

If this sounds like a hippy, New Age fantasy, think again. This deep, indigenous identification with the land is historically normal for the human animal. The bond between body and living habitat is a true human universal and has been taken as self-evident for the vast majority of our time on this planet. As many native people have put it, "I am the land, the land is me" "I am the forest, the forest is me." "I am the river, the river is me." From there, it's but a short step to a job description for the warrior and the artivist: "I'm working for the forest." "I'm working for the ocean, the biosphere, and life on Earth." And ultimately, "We are nature defending herself."

MARTIAL ARTISTRY

Use only that which works, and take it from
any place you can find it.

Bruce Lee
Tao of Jeet Kune Do

A s we've seen, the inactivist avoids conflict whenever
possible goes to great lengths to maintain his neutrality on every issue. He likes to think this orientation
keeps him safe, but it's a fool's errand because conflict is
everywhere in the human experience, as much a part of
our lives as eating and drinking. Hyper-social primates
have some pretty divergent ideas about how to do things
in this world and you won't get far without bumping into
opposition, antagonism, and differences of opinion, if not
outright hostility.

This is especially true in the world of activism. Whenever we seek changes to the status quo it's inevitable that
we'll encounter resistance from those who benefit from
business, government and culture as usual. So what are
we going to do with these conflicted encounters and relationships? The short answer is that we want to prevail but
more to the point, we want to fight skillfully, humanely

and wisely. In other words, we'd like to practice martial art.

But sadly—and sometimes catastrophically—we have almost no training or education in this domain. You probably remember your days as a child and your first encounters with conflict in your neighborhood. If you came from a typical family, Mom said "Don't fight," but Dad said "Don't lose." And schools we're much help in the matter either; it's extremely unlikely that you ever took a course in "Navigating human conflict" at any grade level. Just be nice, stick to the academic work and everything will be OK; so the story went.

And incredibly, that was the end of it—that was the extent of our training for this universal, challenging, and highly consequential human experience. Looking back from the perspective of adulthood and the conflict-related suffering that most of us have had to endure, we might even go so far as to call this a case of educational malpractice. If schools don't prepare us for life and encounters in the real world and the near-term future, what exactly are they doing?

Sadly, this is how most of us have come of age, poorly equipped to deal with this fundamental life experience. It's no wonder that we're awkward, clumsy, and occasionally violent with our bodies and our language, swinging back and forth from one dysfunctional tactic to another. One day we're passive and compliant, but that doesn't work so we swing to impulsive defiance and aggression. That doesn't work either, so we flounder and thrash, avoiding conflict when we can, bluffing our way through the world, sometimes succeeding but mostly just surviving. And in the end, the consequences can be catastrophic; unskillful fighting is expensive, dangerous and counter-productive, both for us and the world around us.

All of which suggests that we'd be better off with some kind of training, or at least some appreciation for martial artistry in a larger sense. But unfortunately, this is where the misunderstanding begins. In the popular imagination, "martial art" is seen as nothing more than spectacular physical skill in hand-to-hand combat, spiced up with occasional nuggets of insight or mysticism. The person who dominates his opponent is honored as the superior fighter, and most importantly, worthy of the silver screen and a million "likes" on social media. But this stereotype severely limits our creativity and sets us up for failure as it obscures the possibilities for real-life success in conflicted relationships, big and small.

To put it another way, our popular, highly visual depictions of martial art action stars distract us from the fact that our most effective conflict artistry is often invisible to the naked eye. Small changes in attitude, spirit, posture, orientation, and attention are fundamental to success in conflicted relationships, but rarely do they appear in visual mediums. In other words, the skills that contribute to effectiveness are subtle, nuanced, and often imperceptible to casual observers. None of which makes for compelling TV, cinema, or YouTube stardom.

A more useful description is to say that martial artistry is about turning conflict into something positive or at least functional. This is actually a common, under-appreciated theme in traditional martial art training. For most teachers, hand-to-hand training is interesting because it gives us valuable metaphors for navigating life as a whole; what traditional teachers often describe as "your practice off the mat." To be sure, personal safety is a real consideration for many people and some hand-to-hand competence makes good sense in certain contexts, but what we're really after is a larger aptitude, a way, an attitude and a presence that can serve us outside the training studio, especially in today's world of radical uncertainty and ambiguity.

The problem, of course, is that most of us have no idea how to show up in this highly conflicted world. A friend suggests that we blockade a road, occupy a bank, organize a march or monkey wrench construction equipment under the cover of darkness. But how do we choose? Do we simply go along with whatever our friends do? What constitutes a good action anyway? How will we know if we've succeeded? What would a seasoned martial artist do in such encounters?

Obviously, there can be no air-tight answers here; activism and martial artistry will never be hard sciences. Every action is different and every artist will have his own opinions. And even more to the point, we're living in unexplored territory now, something that no traditional martial art teacher ever had to deal with. A student might spend decades in rigorous training in a traditional Shaolin Temple and never learn anything about the intricacies of modern politics, law, corporate power, fossil-fueled ecocide, social influence, or organizing.

Nevertheless, there's a wisdom culture here and a tradition of striving for a big picture, systems level intelligence. Traditional teachers understand that physical skill is only a beginning of a more expansive practice. Students must learn the fundamentals of physical movement to be sure, but they're also expected to pay attention to the totality of their predicament and the downstream consequences of their actions. Local victory, by itself, doesn't mean much and might even be a distraction from the larger goal—to touch the world in a sensitive, intelligent, and integrated fashion. So, while the traditional martial art teacher might not be able to tell us precisely what to do in a modern-day activist encounter, he can tell us a great deal about how to show up and what to aspire to.

All of which might seem mystical and esoteric and besides, few of us have the time or opportunity to train in a traditional martial art school. But we already know something about this process via our individual experience. In fact, we can view the entire arc of personal growth and maturity as a martial education in its own right. In other words, what we call "growing up" is a process of learning to exercise good judgment in the face of conflict: learning when to fight, who to fight, what to fight, and especially, how to fight.

Consider the child on the playground, coming to grips with a pushy, belligerent adversary. Other than the standard admonition to "be nice," he really has no idea what to do. Is this fight worth fighting? Should I strike back, run away or say some magic words? With no experience to guide him, he simply reacts impulsively and suffers the consequences. Later, as we mature, our judgment improves, but we continue to waste immense amounts of time and energy fighting the wrong battles, with the wrong people, in the wrong ways.

Finally, after several decades of experience and a few punishing defeats, we become more reflective and selective. We learn to listen to our bodies when they tell us that some situations are best left alone, some are best approached with patience, care, and creativity, and yes, some call for focused, intensive resistance. Our journey to maturity, in other words, is very much a journey to martial artistry. We won't live long enough to perfect the art, but we can develop some useful skills along the way.

OBJECTIVES

So let's start at the beginning, with curiosity and questions. Before exposing ourselves to the challenges and ambiguities of engagement, it's essential that we make a sustained inquiry into methods, targets and objectives. Exactly who or what are we fighting? Are we targeting particular individuals, organizations, policies or legislation? Or are we going after more diffuse objectives such as culture, narratives, or the ideas that flow through the collective unconscious of humanity? What precisely are we trying to do with our time, our energy, and our artivism?

Sadly, many of us never get around to asking these foundational questions. Whipped into a frenzy by the injustices and dysfunctions we see in the world around us, we're quick to go on impulse. Passionate for the cause, we plunge into the work, but before long we become mired in confusion, especially when trying to coordinate with others. Driven by competing visions of an ideal outcome, everyone begins pulling in different directions.

All of which calls for some kind of vision quest, or at least a vision conversation. It might not be necessary to go up on the mountain and fast for several days, but it is essential that we do the work and ask the questions. What's our organization all about? What is this action trying to achieve? What would constitute success? Can we do good *and* feel good in the process?

Start by thinking big. Given the extremity of our predicament, there's simply no time to waste on small-time perpetrators and petty ecological criminals. Instead, go after the biggest offenders within your reach, or even beyond your reach, the true ecocidal maniacs that are wreaking havoc with our world. You can make your own list, but some offenders are obvious: fossil fuel companies and their enablers, corporate apologists and especially, purveyors of anti-future story lines of human supremacy, endless growth, and corporate domination. From there, narrow it down with precision. Which people? Which institutions and companies? Which policies? Which narratives?

Give some thought to your point of focus. Should we concentrate our energies upstream, on the cultural origins of our various afflictions? Or, should we work downstream, at the point of greatest urgency and immediate need? Obviously, downstream issues demand immediate attention; when you've got a hole in your lifeboat, you've got to patch it without delay. But even if you succeed, the original problem remains and you'll probably have to deal with the hole again and again. Maybe it's better to go upstream to the source and deal with whatever caused the hole in the first place. This is why working with young people is so vital. Upstream is where the leverage is.

ENDS AND MEANS

Once you've got an issue and an objective in hand, it's time to organize some kind of action. But what exactly are you going to do? Organize a protest march, hang banners, target financial institutions, or lock yourself down to construction equipment? And what kind of spirit are you going to bring to the action itself? What do you hope to accomplish?

These questions inevitably bring us to the enduring challenge of ends and means. We all have goals and objectives, but how are we to get there? Does it matter what path we take to reach our objective, or is simply achieving the goal enough? What will our martial artistry look like in the process? And most important of all, do the ends justify the means?

Some people will say that in exceptional circumstances—such as our own—the goal is so vital and urgent that it justifies using drastic, even destructive means to get there; just get the job done, no matter what it takes. And at this point in history, it's easy to make just such a case. The urgency and gravity of our predicament is so compelling that we're tempted to say that the end—a functional biosphere—is the only thing that really matters. To put it bluntly, *any* means are now justified. If we fail to protect and preserve the biosphere and atmosphere, there isn't going to *be* a future for the human animal.

If there ever was a case for an ends-over-means justification, this would be it. In our desperation, we're inclined to support any kind of protest, sabotage, disruption, geoengineering, fortress conservation, or even authoritarian military power to save the last remaining shreds of the natural world. It doesn't matter *how* we do it, it just matters *that* we do it.

To put it in the language of athletics, our coach might tell us that winning is now so essential that "winning ugly" is perfectly acceptable. To hell with sportsmanship or any other virtue, this victory is mandatory—if we have to break the rules of fair play along the way, so be it. This is precisely the case explored by Andreas Malm in his 2021 book *How to Blow up a Pipeline.*

In a way, it makes a kind of sense. But then again, it also begs the question "What kind of world do we want to live in?" Ends-over-means might get us the short term survival result we desire, but it also degrades our lives and our experience in the process. When everyone is society lives by ends-over-means thinking, it won't be long before chaos breaks out. In fact, we might well say that an ends-over-means society is really no society at all, just a bunch of primates doing whatever it takes to get what they want.

It's also essential to remember that justifications don't exist in isolation; the thinking that drives the action is always contagious. As hyper-social animals, people pay close attention, not just to the overt behavior of others, but also to the ways that people explain their actions. If the people around us are playing fair and considering the wider world in pursuit of their goals, most of us will imitate their approach. But ugly tactics and an end-over-means attitude will breed more of the same, opening the door to chaos.

Even more to the point, we might well say that the ends-over-means justification is precisely the orientation that got us into this mess in the first place. The end—the modern quest for control, profit and supremacy—is said to justify any sort of behavior, up to and including ecocidal exploitation of the living world. Obviously, adding yet another instance of ends-over-means thinking isn't going to be much of a solution.

All of which is familiar ground in the world of social and spiritual activism, most notably the work of Mahatma Gandhi. As an anti-colonial activist, Gandhi used non-violent resistance to lead the successful campaign for India's independence from British rule. In the process, he took issue with the modern belief in the primacy of ends.

In essence, Gandhi taught that means should be our primary, even exclusive, focus. As he saw it, we cannot get a rose by planting a noxious weed. "The means may be likened to a seed, the end to a tree." Violence and nonviolence are morally different in their essence and will necessarily achieve different results. As he saw it, "Realization of the goal is in exact proportion to that of the means…As the means, so the end."

Likewise, moral philosophers often teach that ends and means are inseparable. Our means—the quality of our actions, our path—should be congruent and consistent with our goals. As Aldous Huxley put it: "Good ends, as I have frequently to point out, can be achieved only by the employment of appropriate means. The end cannot justify the means, for the simple and obvious reason that the means employed determine the nature of the ends produced." In other words, our actions must be crafted, intentionally and consciously, with the process in mind.

Unfortunately, when it comes to the challenge of ends and means, modern culture is pointed precisely in the wrong direction. The last several hundred years has seen a palpable shift towards ends, objectives, and goals—especially bottom-line financial goals at the corporate level. Both individuals and organizations now emphasize results and productivity over almost every other consideration.

In the world of sports, this ends-are-everything obsession was exemplified by football coach Vince Lombardi who famously quipped "Winning isn't everything; it's the only thing." But if Gandhi was an athletic coach, he would have phrased it in the inverse. We might imagine him telling his players to relinquish their focus on outcomes and concentrate instead on quality practice and skill development. As he might have put it, "The means are everything." Or even "Winning is nothing." If you get the process right, the end simply doesn't matter. Or yet again, "The means *are*—or should be—the end."

Ultimately, the most powerful medicine lies in the journey and the quality of the process; we might well say that the medicine is in the means. Even better, focusing on the means can actually make us *more* effective in the long run. Remember, it's all contagious. When people see us showing up with courage, sincerity, resolve, and respect, they'll be inclined to follow along, fighting their battles in a more sophisticated and integrated fashion.

To put it simply, the martial artistry lies in the way we do things. *How* we fight is what matters. Show up over and over again with dignity, integrity, creativity and intent. The victory, you might say, is in the process, not the result.

HARD AND SOFT

Our conversation about ends and means naturally leads us to the issue of tactics and in particular, the differences between hard style and soft style. What kind of force should we bring to a conflict? Is it better to hammer your adversary with focused strikes or blend with the attack and turn it to your advantage? Each style has its place, but it's important to recognize that there are advantages and dangers in both directions.

Hard style includes movements, speech, attitudes, and actions that, in the language of the traditional martial arts, "meet force with force." The power of this approach lies in its clarity and simplicity. The word "No"—in all its various manifestations—sends a clear, unambiguous message: "This is a boundary. You may not cross this boundary. If you cross this boundary, I am going to fight back. You will suffer unpleasant consequences." This kind of action may well be necessary for self-protection, for the defense of people around us or our life-support systems. When used appropriately, it's a useful, practical, functional skill.

If you happen to choose a hard style response, commitment is vital. Whether it's verbal, physical, or even symbolic, it's important to be clear about where your boundaries lie. When you make the decision to act, don't waver. Speak with conviction and confidence, backed up by assertive body language and posture. If under physical assault, use a *kiai*, the high-energy shout used in traditional martial arts. Bring all your psychophysical resources together into a single, integrated, and powerful act.

But, of course, hard style responses aren't always appropriate, especially when they're impulsive. When we become angry or fearful, we lose our sense of proportion, and in the extreme, our hard style responses can turn ugly. When we fight fire with fire, things tend to escalate and it's all wickedly contagious. In the process, you may well inspire your adversary and bystanders to increase their resistance and retaliate. Even if you happen to win a particular encounter, you've inflamed the system and increased the chances that you'll have to suffer hard style actions coming back the other way.

A better choice might be a *soft style* response in which we "use the enemy's strength against him." This is the guiding principle in the practice of *aikido, judo* and several other arts. If you can amplify or exaggerate your opponents' movement, you can lead him out of balance, into a state of instability. From there it becomes easy—in theory at least—to turn his movement into a fall or pin him to the ground.

The quintessential expressions of this soft-style approach come from the Taoist tradition, most notably Lao-tzu in his classic work, the *Tao Te Ching*:

> The highest good is like water... Nothing in the world is softer and weaker than water. Yet there is nothing better for subduing all that is harder and stronger.

> What you want to compress you must first truly allow to expand. What you want to weaken you must first allow to grow strong. What you want to destroy you must first allow to truly flourish. From whoever you want to take away, you must first truly give. This is called being clear about the invisible. The soft wins victory over the hard. The weak wins victory over the strong.

In conversation or political discourse, you might think of this soft-style approach as *hyperagreement*. Instead of opposing your adversary's positions, encourage his extremity. Blend with his language; amplify and exaggerate his ideas. As Sun Tzu put it in *The Art of War*, "Pretend inferiority and encourage his arrogance." Help him take his opinions, movements, and actions to the point of absurdity and, in turn, reversal. At some point, he'll either realize his folly or lapse into a state of frustration and confusion.

It's a seductive idea and in some cases, it can be a practical, effective solution. It might even be useful when a smaller and weaker David goes up against a vastly more powerful Goliath. The beauty of this approach is that—if executed with a high level of skill—it doesn't inflame or provoke a counter-reaction. When perfectly executed, your opponent essentially throws himself.

But there are substantial caveats and real dangers here. If you're too soft in your response or fail to maintain an integrated posture, you may well be overwhelmed. If you misread your adversary's intentions or fail to turn his movement to your advantage, all may be lost.

In fact, the soft-style approach requires an exceptionally high level of training, skill, understanding, and attention. If you want to use your adversary's movements against him, you've got to know precisely what he's doing and what he's trying to accomplish. This suggests that you've got to be a dedicated student of your adversary, his history, his values, and ideology. What moves your opponent? What are his objectives? What's his stance and position? What's the trajectory of his behavior? The more understanding you have, the better. Once you know your adversary's intentions and inclinations, you're in a better position to help him go to self-defeating extremes.

Likewise, soft style also calls for a spirit of non-attachment and psycho-spiritual flexibility. To execute a successful blend, you've got to abandon your personal likes and dislikes, at least for the time being. Read your adversaries, get inside their minds, relinquish your position and adopt their movements as your own. The more complete your blend, the easier it will be to nudge them in a new direction.

Naturally, people are quick to argue about the relative

merits of hard and soft styles, and some will claim that one is superior to the other. But out in the real world, the martial artist must be versatile and capable of both. Our adversaries are in a constant state of flux, and it's hard to predict what they might do. If all you've got is one style, you're going to be limited, ineffective, and, ultimately, vulnerable.

In other words, it's best to be ambidextrous and enter each encounter with a sense of balance and equipoise. You've got a plan and an objective, but you're ready and willing to change your movement and your intent on the fly. If soft doesn't work, be ready for something more direct. If hard doesn't work, turn down the heat and see if a blend might be more effective.

NON-PARTICIPATION

There's yet another layer to this art. Most of us are quick to think of martial art as something we do, fighting off the forces of evil, resolving disputes, or making something beautiful out of conflicted situations. We engage the opposition and prevail by way of our superior skills, knowledge, creativity, or wits.

But we might also do well to think of martial artistry as something we *don't* do. In this practice, we step aside and disengage with people, institutions, and processes that are harmful to the future, society and the planet. By withholding our participation, we make these systems weaker.

All of which reminds us of the old quip "What if they gave a war and nobody came?" It's a great question because it forces us to consider the fact that participation in toxic systems is not inevitable; we can choose another path. Social pressure to conform is real, but at our core, we're nothing but a bunch of primates. The hawks tell us that military action is inevitable and that everyone must line up, but if we don't participate, the effort loses its power, energy and legitimacy. In fact, the war is only possible because vast numbers of people are obedient and willing to comply

Likewise, we might well put our question in modern, ecological terms: "What if they gave a planetary house wrecking party and no one came?" What if people simply refused to participate in toxic industries? What if people simply stopped participating in new fossil fuel projects, plastic production, industrial logging, industrial agriculture, and industrial fishing? What if people refused to participate in the marketing and advertising of useless consumer junk? What if people stopped participating in the glorification of wealth? And most important of all, what if people stopped valuing the kind of lifestyle that is sold to us as the only possible way to live?

The consequences would be swift and world changing. Just imagine if corporate multi-nationals could no longer find workers to build their monstrosities. What if they could no longer find people to cut down forests, build pipelines, maintain industrial agriculture, or finance and insure their mega-projects? Change would come in a heartbeat.

Obviously, there are substantial personal risks involved in this kind of strategy. Follow your conscience and you may well find yourself struggling to make ends meet and you may have to fall back on your creative powers to get by. It's also the case that there are plenty of judgment calls involved. It's not always easy to say precisely which kinds of participation are most destructive. In fact, many modern corporations are ethical hybrids, which is to say, they've got one foot in beneficial products and services, and the other in planet-killing enterprises.

There's plenty of uncertainty and exposure that comes with non-participation and you might well find yourself disconnected from familiar sources of support and certainty, but that ambiguity is nothing compared to the inevitability of chaos and destruction that comes with giving our time and energy to a mindless, planet-devouring mechanism. Withdraw your support and you might suffer in transition; maintain your support and you're certain to go down with the ship. So stop giving the machine the fuel that it needs. Walk away and let it die.

CREATIVE DISRUPTION

For aspiring martial artists in the modern world, one of the most interesting inquiries has to do with the nature of society and in particular, the origins of our large-scale dysfunctions. Why is it that so many of us have come to participate in systems that are inherently toxic, both to people and the natural world? What are the psycho-spiritual conditions that make atrocity possible?

According to many scholars, the problem begins with obedience itself. Compliance with authority does have a role to play in social harmony and function, but it's equally true that obedience has a nasty, highly destructive shadow side. In fact, obedience can pave the way for all manner of violence—to other human beings and even to the planet as a whole.

The most obvious example comes to us via the work of social psychologist Stanley Milgram, described in his legendary work *Obedience to Authority*. As Milgram discovered, human beings can be incredibly compliant in the face of authority and will even over-ride their personal moral sensibilities and judgment. When a white-coated authority figure demands that we perform a task that will hurt other people, we're likely to do as we're told.

This sets the stage for all manner of bad behavior. As Milgram concluded, "The essence of obedience consists in the fact that a person comes to view himself as the instrument for carrying out another person's wishes. He therefore no longer regards himself as responsible for his actions." In other words, the obedient person is no longer an activist or an artivist, but simply an agent for someone else's plans and vision.

Milgram's work focused primarily on obedience in interpersonal relationships, but we can be sure that obedience also has destructive consequences in the domain of habitat destruction and other future-hostile behaviors. Industrial agriculture, industrial fishing, deforestation, mining, and fossil fuel development all require large organizations, staffed with compliant workers and managers who dutifully carry out their orders. It's impossible to measure, but we can be certain that a large proportion of ecocidal behavior is only possible because of obedient workers. As the street artist Banksy put it, "The greatest crimes in the world are not committed by people breaking the rules but by people following the rules."

THE ART OF DISOBEDIENCE

So what's to be done? Nearly every informed activist now believes that revolutionary, systemic transformation is the only viable path to a functional future. Conventional protests and polite appeals to power simply aren't working, As the youth activists of Climate Defiance put it, "We tried being polite, and it didn't work." Likewise, Marianne Williamson, "The system will not disrupt itself." And author Chris Hedges: "Civil disruption is all we have left."

So it's time to create some trouble—especially what civil rights activist John Lewis called "good trouble." This is a call for nonviolent civil disobedience, the intentional disruption of business, government, and culture-as-usual. The value of this practice is that it disturbs the flow of power in society and public perceptions about what may or may not be ethically acceptable. As Martin Luther King, Jr., put it, the objective is to "dramatize the conflict so that it can no longer be ignored."

Captain Paul Watson, formerly of the Sea Shepherd Conservation Society, has blockaded and harassed whalers and factory fisheries on the open seas for years, in a practice he calls "aggressive nonviolence." For Watson, the goal is to "...obstruct, intervene, interfere, harass... accepting risk, getting in the face of adversaries, and calling out their crimes, but never engaging in violence to humans or non-human nonhuman animals."

It's hard to say how effective these tactics are, but the biggest benefit may actually be indirect. Civil disobedience may not substantially change the immediate behavior of your adversary, but it will communicate to others the seriousness of your resolve and your willingness to take risks for the sake of the future. It also shifts the Overton window of acceptable discourse and in turn, behavior. When people speak out and stand up, it normalizes the practice and changes public opinion.

This is why attitude, stance, and spirit are so important.

Bystanders will witness your tree-sit, your road blockade, or your lockdown at a bank or government office. They'll be curious about your position on the issue in question, but even more important, they'll be alert for the tone and tenor of your message, especially your sincerity. In this sense, the details of your action are less important than the dignity and resolve that you bring to the doing. This is why civil disobedience more than just trouble-making; in essence, it's a deeply spiritual practice.

PROPERTY DESTRUCTION?

Nonviolence is obviously an essential practice and must be at the heart of every action, but as to questions about property destruction, that's another matter entirely. When we've tried everything else, what's left but to destroy the physical end points of fossil-fueled domination: the mining equipment, the drilling and fracking equipment, and the private jets that ferry ecocidal elites from place to place?

This suggestion will strike conventionalists as extreme, but their argument is flawed. How is it that we sanction the overt, intentional, mechanized, and automated destruction of habitat and life itself, and yet criminalize damage to the machines that cause that destruction? In essence, industrial culture prioritizes the exploitation of the natural world while criminalizing anything that gets in the way. One is declared "progress," the other is labeled "felony vandalism."

And just to be clear, the destruction of future-hostile machinery is not violence. In fact, the whole point is to *prevent* further violence against habitat, people, animals, and the future. Destruction of life is violence; destruction of life-hostile machines is an act of protection of the innocent and the powerless; done properly, it's an act of self-defense.

To be sure, simple tools and even modest machinery can be life-enhancing and maybe even sustainable in some way, but beyond the point of optima they become ugly, toxic and deserving of destruction. There's a very real difference between a broom and a leaf blower, between a bicycle and an SUV. There's a very real difference between a small fishing boat that takes a few salmon by line and a factory supertrawler that sucks up every living thing in its path. One is appropriate, romantic and life-enhancing; the other is simply ugly. One should be celebrated and preserved; the other deserves whatever it gets.

CULTURAL MONKEY WRENCHES

But the destruction of property, even in its most appropriate and creative forms, isn't really going to move the needle on the world. Future-hostile enterprises have extremely deep pockets, are massively insured, and highly motivated to continue their work. Taking out a few bulldozers isn't going to slow them down.

But perhaps we can be more effective by working at a higher level, taking on the upstream ideas and cultural assumptions that drive the Earth-hostile practices in the first place. For example, consider the disruptive potential of these cultural monkey wrenches:

- Bioregionalism, the re-drawing of political boundaries to reflect actual life conditions on the ground.

- Wild law and rights of nature, in which we shift the focus away from anthropocentrism to be more inclusive of life as a whole.

- Ecocide law, in which we re-define criminal behavior to reflect actual harm to habitat and future generations.

- Corporate charter revision, in which society re-writes corporate law to demand social and ecological responsibility. This would include the elimination of tax havens and a Robin Hood tax on stock transactions.

- True cost pricing, whereby the cost that's listed for our various products and services reflects the actual cost to habitat and humanity.

- The Paleo/indigenous world view: the historically-normal cluster of ideas that includes interdependence, continuity, reciprocity, animism, oral tradition, bioregionalism, and *ubuntu* (identification with tribe and people).

No matter the details, all these proposals call for big shifts in the Overton window of acceptable discourse. The mere act of talking and writing about these proposals opens up new possibilities and sheds light on the deep assumptions of modern culture. In other words, your keyboard and your voice matter. Monkeywrench the dominant cultural narratives of our age and you might well inspire real change.

WHAT COMES NEXT?

Non-violent civil disobedience and cultural monkey-wrenching sound promising, but there's one more consideration that deserves our attention; the often-ignored question "What comes next?" When confronted with monstrous injustice, criminality, and systemic dysfunction, our first impulse is often to simply tear down the entire toxic system. The ecocidal-social injustice machine is ripping the planet to shreds and it must be stopped. Conventional measures have failed and now it's time to bring the entire dysfunctional system to a grinding halt.

All of which feels perfectly understandable and just. But then what? Society abhors a vacuum we might say, so who or what's going to step into the gap? When we tear down existing systems of governance, law, and policy, we create openings for every hack, grifter, opportunist, and would-be tyrant who might be waiting in the wings. And in the long run, we might well make things worse.

All of which calls for a strategy of creative disruption, coupled with active building up of viable alternatives. In other words, a tearing down *and* a building up. For every act of rebellion, some act of creation. Call this the yin and yang of creative disruption: For every no, a yes; for every act of resistance, an act of vision and imagination. Disrupt the system, absolutely, but give people something to do and believe in on the other side.

NARRATIVE ACTIVISM

Most of us think of martial art as something we do with our fists and feet, but in the larger sense, it's really about our fluency with language, ideas, and in particular, the power of story.

In fact, story is one of the most potent forces in the human experience. Story holds the master ideas of a culture, gives us a sense of priority and helps us navigate the tough judgment calls that we face each day. The beauty of story is that it bypasses rational, cognitive labor and appeals directly to the human imagination.

Sadly, the state of story in the modern world is chaos. Once a powerful force for cultural focus and meaning, story has devolved into a means of passive entertainment and, of course, profit. Over the last several decades, we've grown accustomed to the notion that the primary purpose of story is to keep us amused and even distracted. A story is considered "good" if it keeps our attention for the duration of the telling, and if it "captures eyeballs," as the marketers put it, so much the better.

All of which is historically unprecedented. In the Paleolithic world of hunting and gathering, story was absolutely critical to survival and tribal function. People coalesced around a small number of narratives, repeated often. Stories explained the world and held people together; everyone in your tribe would have known the master narratives. You heard the stories almost every night and slept well, secure in the knowledge that life made some kind of coherent sense.

But today we're suffering from an avalanche of fragmented narratives, each describing some narrow facet of reality or the human experience, and all of them competing with one another for the last remaining fragments of our attention. Today we have an astronomical number of stories, but they come and go with the digital wind, and rarely do they hang around long enough to bring us together.

Even worse, our modern storytelling landscape is populated by a glut of plastic, synthetic narratives; inauthentic, artificial nuggets of guidance about how to live, brought to us by corporate marketing departments. These faux life lessons are massively premeditated, focus-group-tested and produced. They tell us how to look, train, work, love, value, and experience life. Like fast food, these hyper-refined narratives are easy to consume, but displace the authentic human stories that we so desperately need.

So what's to be done? Conditioned by conventional culture, many activists are quick to assume that the only way to make a difference is through the use of political power and social force. Get the right academic degree, go to law school, ascend to the right government or corporate position, and start wielding power. But no matter your rank in a hierarchy, story remains essential. Crafting and sharing the right narrative at the right time can make the difference between failure and success. In fact, story is implicit in everything we do as activists. No matter the details of our protests, blockades, or civil disobedience, there's always a set of assumptions and expectations that's wrapped up in the doing. In this sense, *all* activism is—or should be—narrative in nature.

All of which begs the question: How do we wield our narrative powers? How do we talk to the media, to our audiences, and to people who might have some leverage? How should we talk to our allies and our adversaries? Obviously, you'd like your listeners to hear your story and maybe even adopt your perspective on the issue in question, but before you put your fingers to the keyboard or sit yourself down in front of a webcam, it's essential to circle back and review your methods and your objectives...

TELL THE TRUTH

Begin with the first principle of Extinction Rebellion: "Tell the truth." Give people the scientific facts and trajectories as you understand them. Don't sugar coat the predicament or offer false hope. Speak to the urgency of the moment but be thoughtful with your tone. Are you painting an apocalyptic picture of an imminent, inevitable global disaster or are you offering a pathway forward?

Obviously, conditions are desperate, but adding another layer of fear and panic to the mix is unlikely to be helpful. To be sure, some people need to feel the heat and in particular, inactvists and perpetrators need to understand the extremity of the situation. If we can turn up the pressure with scientific facts, maybe they'll be moved to action.

But for many readers and listeners, it all goes the other way. Many people already understand the gravity of our predicament and if we subject them to yet more angst, they might just shut down and revert to the familiar. So of course it's a judgment call. People do need to feel a sense of urgency, but they also need to feel a sense of *agency*. Yes, tell the truth, but give people some power and control to work with. Instead of intensifying fear, speak of promise, possibility, opportunity that lies in participation and engagement. Remind people of the power and medicinal qualities of activism. Win or lose, activism is good for you.

SAY NO TO PASSIVE VOICE

A closely-related truth-telling practice is to stop using passive voice to describe criminal and ecocidal behavior. Stop saying that "mistakes were made." Stop saying "The

Earth is heating up," "The forest was clear-cut," "The atmosphere was poisoned" or "Species were driven to extinction." Passive voice makes it sound as if these events simply happened spontaneously, maybe even by accident. This is what comedian George Carlin would have ridiculed as "soft language."

In fact, in most of these cases, there are actual agents involved; perpetrators, people, cultures, and organizations making conscious, intentional, even criminal decisions. These actors, whether they be individuals or organizations, have names and must be called out. The problem with passive voice is that it contributes to what's called "social license," an implicit approval granted by our habits of speech. Whenever possible, point to the perpetrators with active voice; a person or organization did something or is doing something.

BEWARE MILITANT LANGUAGE

At the same time, it's important to be careful with militant language and military metaphors. In our passion for change, we're often inclined to see everything through the lenses of conflict, opposition, and extremes; a thing is either this way or that way, you're either with us or against us. Everyone is either an ally or an adversary, a force for good or a force for evil. There's no middle ground, no hybrids, and no complementary relationships.

To be sure, militant language can feel good and sometimes has its place, but it can also lead to premature polarization by forcing people into corners and pigeonholes. This inflames relationships that might actually be on their way to resolution. Militant language over-simplifies complex realities and can even polarize things unnecessarily. When your language destroys the middle ground, it can be hard to go back.

Even worse, militant language is extremely contagious. Every time we hear polarizing statements, we're more likely to adopt similar black-and-white perspectives. And in short order, everyone is locked into either-or orientations, which only increases the adversarial energy in the system. Is this what you want? Do you really want to force a highly complex reality into a polarized, adversarial form? Maybe it's better to save the militant language as a last resort.

"YES, AND..."

Even better, it also helps to consider the way we respond to one another in conversation. As you've probably noticed, our modern, oppositional minds are quick to refute, rebut, and attack, all of which is contained in language that begins with the word "But..." Not surprisingly, this gets things off to a bad start as the word negates whatever came before it. "But..." nullifies, rejects, discards, and diminishes. We can even be sure that there's a neuro-psychological effect with this kind of language; as soon as we hear the word "But" most of us are quick to fire up our oppositional cognition and go on the defensive.

A more promising approach is to nurture relationships and a sense of possibility by using the "Yes, and..." construction. Suddenly, everything changes. Opponents, or potential opponents feel heard, validated, and even felt. "Yes, I understand your perspective and I understand the history behind your views, and I'd like to propose an additional way of looking at our predicament." It's not a perfect solution or cure-all for disagreement, but it does clear a path to some kind of future. Things may still be murky or stressful, but now we can feel a sense of potential, a possibility for resolution. In other words, "Yes, and" can be a profoundly creative act of martial artistry.

HEAD AND HEART

It's also important to leverage the humanities and speak in the language of the body, which is to say, the heart. As veteran social justice activist David Fenton teaches, "speak to the heart first, the mind second." Unfortunately, this is where many highly educated speakers go astray. As professor George Lakoff points out, many of us—especially in university culture—are trained to believe that facts are persuasive on their own. We may even come to look down on the idea of selling ideas through metaphor or imagery. Lakoff calls this "the enlightenment fallacy."

Consultants in the world of public speaking make a similar observation, as author Randy Olson points out in his book *Don't Be Such a Scientist*. As Olson sees it, scientists are trained to use a particular style of language with a particular mission: the transmission and presentation of methods, findings and data. The facts are supposed to speak for themselves, but most people outside the university community don't listen this way. In fact, most humans are moved first and foremost by feeling. This is why highly educated scientists and academics are often at a disadvantage in the domain of public persuasion.

All of which suggests that if we're going to be effective, we need to avoid the disembodied, Cartesian speaking style that puts data front and center. These presentations do serve a specialized purpose, but are death to public persuasion. Graphs, charts, and mathematical equations only work for people trained in that domain. For everyone else, they feel more like a form of punishment.

THE ENEMY IS NEVER WRONG

Finally, it's essential that we look back to our spirit and our mind-set as martial artists. Whenever we engage in conflict at any level, we enter into what's been called "the fog of war." Conditions are always changing, enemies are devious, and unknown agents and processes can wreak havoc with our best-laid plans.

In this uncertain and dynamic world, physical flexibility is an asset, but even more important is our psycho-spiritual orientation and especially, the way we relate to our experience. In turn, this becomes a vital question for martial artists and activists: Am I working from a place of resistance or acceptance?

On the face of it, resistance would seem to be the name of the game. Someone has violated a boundary, assaulted us physically or attacked someone or something we care about or identify with—including habitat and the Earth at large. That person or organization must be stopped with direct action. We need a forceful response, backed up by a psycho-spiritual attitude of resistance and even enmity. The enemy is wrong and we're out to make things right again.

All of which sounds perfectly sensible and appropriate. Fighting back is often necessary, honorable, and maybe even sapient. Nevertheless, there's danger here. In our resistance, we may well become consumed by our antagonism and in the process, loose our sense of fluidity, movement, and adaptability.

The challenge of combat is that adversaries don't just threaten our bodies, loved ones, and values, they also capture our minds. Their behavior strikes us as outrageous; they have no right to behave the way they do, no justification for their actions or their attitude. They must be crazy or evil or both. In the process, our emotion begins to tyrannize our consciousness and our imagination. Our adversaries don't just threaten our welfare; they also send us into vicious cycles of fear, projection, rumination, obsession, and demonizing. Before long, our performance collapses and we become ineffective, or worse.

This is why traditional martial art teachers often advise their students to turn their minds around and consider the possibility that "the enemy is never wrong." This counsel may well sound surprising and even preposterous on its face, but the lesson is both sound and relevant to the challenges of our age. The idea is to remain fluid and adaptable in the face of adversity—don't get wrapped up in some expectation about what your situation should or shouldn't be. Abandon your psychic resistance, at least for the moment; your opponent, your predicament just is. Fight for what you believe in, but don't get caught up in unnecessary judgment and evaluation. Don't be trapped by your own mind.

This is not to say we should simply accept everything about the world as it is. Of course the destruction of our biosphere is wrong and must be opposed. Of course fossil fuel companies are perpetrators of criminal ecocide. Of course the exploitation and domination of other people is wrong and must be called out. Rather, this is an argument for radical realism and adaptability. It's about letting go of expectation and working with the world as it presents itself. When we adopt this point of view, our indignation, anxiety, and stress become optional, or at least less tyrannical. You may still struggle and suffer, but you'll see things more clearly. Your experience and your effectiveness will improve substantially and in the long run, "the enemy is never wrong" might well be the ultimate koan for stress relief, resilience, and adaptive psychology.

The value in this kind of detachment is that it allows us to see our opponents clearly, without prejudice, expectation, or prediction. Our adversaries are unpredictable agents who are capable of anything, so the less we assume about them the better. That's why the ideal response is fluidity in motion—pure creativity, pure adaptability, and pure improv. Bruce Lee himself argued for maximum flexibility in combat, and even created his own martial art form: *Jeet Kune Do*, the "style of no style."

> Empty your mind...be formless, shapeless, like water. If you put water into a cup, it becomes the cup. You put water into a bottle and it becomes the bottle. You put it in a teapot, it becomes the teapot. Now water can flow, or it can crash. Be water, my friend.

This all makes good sense in the world of hand-to-hand martial artistry but is even more powerful when we apply it to the totality of our life experience. What if we practiced this kind of emotional detachment on a larger scale? Just imagine a life in which...

People are never wrong.

Culture is never wrong.

Events are never wrong.

Laws and policies are never wrong.

Your emotions are never wrong.

The people in your life are never wrong.

Your anxiety, stress, and depression are never wrong.

Your injuries and illnesses are never wrong.

Looking at the world this way, the rightness or wrongness of your situation would be irrelevant and, in turn, powerless to distract you. You'd be free to see clearly and act effectively, without friction, stress, resistance, or anxiety.

To be sure, this perspective can never be easy, pure, or absolute, nor would we want it to be. We are emotional animals after all, and we're sensitive to injustices of all kinds. We want life to be fair and we're quick to react, sometimes powerfully and passionately, to negative events, especially those we consider unjust. Sometimes our bodies respond instinctively, driven by ancient, legacy programming beyond the reach of conscious control. It would be nonhuman—even nonanimal—to stand completely apart from life and view it all with cold objectivity.

Nevertheless, a little detachment can go a long way. Can you pause and step back, even for a moment? Can you see your predicament without judgment or expectation? Can you adopt the perspective of a scientist or a journalist and see the thing in question just as it is? Take a breath, relax, and imagine no judgment.

Just to be clear, this is not an argument for apathy, passivity, or an uncritical acceptance of everything in the world. Some things on this planet are wickedly, morally wrong and must be opposed with all the power we can muster. Fighting remains essential, honorable, and sapient. We must never forget the atrocities that have been committed and that continue to be perpetrated on people, animals, and the planet. The historical memory of such events is truly sacred.

Nevertheless, this "never wrong" approach is highly functional. The sooner we accept the reality of negative events, ideas, people, and experiences, the sooner we can get to work devising effective strategies and tactics. Radical realism leaves preference and expectation behind. Let go of the angst; deal with reality and your adversary without illusion. Observe, relax, then move.

Remember, life is capable of anything. People are capable of anything. Humans are highly complex, irrational animals, struggling to live in an alien, highly stressful environment. We'd all like to have things a certain way, but our preferences are not the issue. Our job is to create and re-create adaptations on the fly. If we can let go of our indignation, we can start fresh and return to the encounter with a clear vision.

STRESS

There are enough real enemies and threats in the world without having to invent imaginary ones.

Christina Engela
Dead Man's Hammer

Activism, artivism, martial art—all these practices bring us into conflict with entrenched individuals, ideas, organizations and institutions that are opposed or even hostile to change. When we try to change any-thing—much less the entire trajectory of the industrial-ized world—we're going to face resistance, friction, and stress. If we're going to get anything done, it's essential that we understand how this experience affects our bodies, our cognition and our behavior, as well as the bodies, cogni-tion, and behavior of our allies and adversaries.

The place to begin is by understanding the breadth and depth of the challenge. Put simply, modern humans are laboring under a monstrous, crushing stress burden, un-precedented in human history, and the consequences, both personal and social, are severe. To be sure, humans have always experienced stress in various forms, some-times acute, sometimes chronic, but today's stressors are almost diabolical in their novelty, diversity, and ferocity.

Our hunting and gathering ancestors were stressed by wild animals, wildfires, bad weather, conflicts with other tribes and occasional disease and injury, but they also found comfort in an integrative life experience and continuity with the natural world. Life was harsh at times, but it was also filled with awe and simple comforts. Even better, stress was experienced socially and rhythmically; go on a hunt, chase or be chased, activate your fight-flight system, then return to camp for a few days of rest, food, and gossip. This oscillation is ideal for autonomic health, cognition, and performance.

In contrast, today's stressors are novel, often intense, and grindingly chronic. Even the list itself is anxiety-provoking: looming ecological collapse, social and economic inequality, pandemics that come and go, hyper-normal stimuli and mixed sensory messages, radical increases in complexity and unpredictability, social polarization, misinformation and declines in social trust, cognitive overload (every little thing is a homework project), temporal poverty (never enough time), random violence, economic uncertainty, a hyper-competitive, winner-take-all culture, political gridlock, social media (conflict and comparison on demand), and worst of all, no apparent endpoint to any of it.

Incredibly, much of this burden was foreshadowed by Alvin Toffler's 1970 book *Future Shock* in which he described our affliction as "too much change in too short a period of time." In other words, the hockey stick of accelerating change is wreaking havoc, not just on the biosphere, but on the entire human mind-body-social system; the human organism can only take so much dynamism and ambiguity before it breaks down.

To make matters worse, we're also extremely confused about the sources of our stress and incredibly, we don't even agree on what's dangerous in our world. And if we're not sure what's dangerous, we're not going to be stressed out about the right things, at the right time and in the right degree. This is a recipe for disaster and in turn, more stress.

Just take a look at human history: For most of our time on earth, the fundamental physical threats were obvious to everyone, even children: large animals, snakes, wildfires, raging rivers, gravity (high places), and on some occasions, neighboring tribes. The challenges were easy to feel and comprehend, our stress was coherent and even better, people could come to an easy consensus about what to do, where to go, and how to live. When people understand and agree on dangers, they experience a shared state of *autonomic cohesion*. When everyone in your tribe is experiencing a similar degree of fight-flight or rest-and-digest, it's just a whole lot easier to get along.

Fast forward a few millennia to the modern age. Beginning with the scientific and industrial revolution, we experienced a burst of innovation, much of it welcome and beneficial, but with every new technology, novel and often incomprehensible dangers came along for the ride— dangers that are utterly unfamiliar and sometimes even invisible to the naked eye: strange chemicals in our food and water, fine print in contracts, computer viruses, data breaches, phishing and now quishing attacks (QR code scams), AI, unknowable fluctuations in financial markets, strange new legal and social relationships between people, and worst of all perhaps, a sense of alienation from the living world.

This multiplication of stressors has amplified our stress a thousand-fold and to make matters even worse, has led to a radically fractured human experience, a state of *autonomic incoherence*. Just imagine the people on a modern city street, each one absorbed in their various dramas and challenges. In all likelihood, these individuals will have very different opinions about what's dangerous. Some will be near panic, in a heightened state of fight-flight-freeze; others will be easing into a state of rest-and-digest or feed-and-breed. With so much autonomic diversity in play, it becomes almost impossible to work together. If we can't agree on what's dangerous, how are we supposed to reach consensus on practical matters? And naturally, all this confusion feeds back on itself to amplify our stress burden even further.

THE ENCOUNTER

All of which gives us an important starting point for our work as activists and martial artists: the recognition that modern humans are deep in the psycho-spiritual red zone. In other words, it makes sense to simply assume stress and trauma in ourselves and the people we encounter each day. Their struggles may not be overt or obvious, but as physicians Gabor Mate and Bessel van der Kolk have made abundantly clear, these afflictions are widespread and might even amount to a modern human universal. It's safe to assume that most of the people we come in contact with—allies and adversaries alike—will be suffering some combination of loss, cognitive overload, trauma, grief and existential angst.

And of course, the consequences of this burden go far beyond individual health. We've all heard a great deal about personal susceptibility to various lifestyle diseases, decreased athletic performance, and premature aging, but it's actually worse than all that. Stress also has a wide array of collective and social consequences, *all* of them working against our efforts to create a functional future: reversion to the familiar, siege mentality and hoarding, reactivity and impulsivity, xenophobia and incivility, displaced aggression, learned helplessness, cynicism and despair, compassion fatigue, decision fatigue, diminished curiosity, and most notoriously, inactivism. Worst of all, stress and fear drive out our best human attributes—compassion, creativity, empathy—the very qualities that we desperately need at this moment in history.

All of which adds up to a compelling, urgent need for public stress education. With so many tigers—both real and false—circling our camp, we've got to learn how to take care of our bodies and our spirits. This training is vital, not just for activism, but for our very ability to survive and function in today's alien environment. To be sure, some educational programs do exist, but much work remains to be done. In fact, stress is so destructive to the modern human experience that stress education must be considered absolutely vital to the creation of a functional future. If we can't get our stress under control, it's unlikely that we'll make much progress on the atmosphere or the biosphere either.

KNOW THE BEAST

But what exactly is this thing we call "stress?" Most of us

understand it as a toxic feeling, a personal experience in our bodies and our minds. Time pressure, relational turmoil, money woes, problems at work; all of it coming together in a cluster of unpleasant sensation; muscles tighten, thoughts race, patience wears thin, outlook contracts. We may not have words to describe it, but we know it when we feel it.

In the scientific world, researchers tell us that stress is triggered by "a perceived threat to the organism," but this only tells us so much. Yes, perception and interpretation are essential to our experience and the functioning of our bodies, but there's a lot more to the story. In fact, stress can be triggered by a wide range of influences:

- A perceived loss of control over our circumstances, our work, our social standing, our bodies, our future.

- Too much novelty in too little time; radical acceleration of change beyond our ability to adapt.

- A loss of connection; especially connections to our social life-supporting systems of family, friends, and colleagues.

- A loss of coherence; especially the feeling that our world no longer makes sense.

Taken all around, this sounds like a fitting description of the modern world itself. Radical acceleration and breathtaking increases in complexity erode our sense of control and our sense of coherence. Couple this with isolation and a loss of connection, and you're likely to suffer a serious, even debilitating stress burden.

OBJECTIVES

So what's to be done with these stressful experiences and sensations? In conventional conversations, most people assume that since stress is an unpleasant experience, our goal is simply to make it go away; in other words, a stress-free life is the ideal. Across the popular press, this is the simplistic message we see on magazine covers and websites everywhere—utopian promises to help us lead a "stress-free life" and "banish stress forever."

All of which may seem appealing in the moment, but on reflection, we're inclined to wonder. What if stress is actually important information? What if it's telling us something vital about our lives? What if it's helping to keep us safe and alive? If that's the case, do we really want to "banish stress forever?"

Suppose your physician or therapist offers you a formula—a medication, procedure, or an exercise that promises to eliminate your stress. Would you take it? And if it actually worked, then what? You'd be feeling great, but the planet and its inhabitants would still be suffering, the wounds would still exist. In this respect, our aspiration to live without stress would be a fool's goal; a stress-free life would also be a life of irrelevance.

The problem is that most of the time, especially at this moment in history, stress just isn't that articulate. Sometimes it's telling us a very clear and coherent story about the lions and tigers in our lives, but other times it just sort of grinds away at our minds, not really telling us precisely what's wrong. And it's enormously difficult to sort it all out. Some of our stress feels meaningful, important, and worthy of our attention, but some of it—most of it perhaps—we could just as well do without.

All of which challenges us to be better listeners of our experience, to pay closer attention to functional and dysfunctional stress sensations. Instead of simply trying to make stress "go away," a better objective is to be sensitive and responsive to the right stressors, in the right degree, at the right time. To put it another way, we need to become fluent in our relationship to stress, to understand what it's telling us and respond appropriately.

STRESS EDUCATION

In turn, this brings us back to stress education and what we might call "the use and abuse of the autonomic nervous system." The first thing to understand is that in one sense, it's actually pretty easy to make our stress go away. Just shut down awareness of the offending person, process, experience, or event, and magically, you'll feel better, at least for a while. If something causes you angst, cognitive overload or moral confusion, just look in some other direction and presto—problem solved.

It's a common strategy of course and probably even a human universal. No one wants to focus on the things in life that suggest a loss of control or coherence; all of us would rather stay in the sweet spot of pleasant, comforting experience. But this is precisely the problem that we see in the domain of climate and ecological destruction. It hurts to look at the devastation of the Earth and the injustices in society, so we look away, into the world of amusement, entertainment, and pleasure. This is the "strategy" practiced by millions of people around the world, facilitated and encouraged by pleasure-centric marketing and advertising.

But in the long run, this distortion of attention—this willful blindness—will wreak havoc with our life experience. You can look away from the lions and tigers and bears if you choose, but your life will begin to lose its relevance and even its meaning. And the predators will still be out there, and they'll still be hungry. It may be unpleasant to keep your eyes open, but it's better for all of us in the long run.

KNOW THE CURVE

The next thing to understand is that contrary to the standard narrative, stress is not always bad for us. The popular press tells us that stress is uniformly nasty; it makes us more susceptible to disease, causes premature aging, destroys our sexual vitality and our athletic performance, and even degrades the tissues of our brains. Some of us even come to live in fear of stress and do everything in our power to make it go away.

But this narrative ignores the fact that in small or moderate doses, stress is incredibly beneficial to the entire mind-body system. It sharpens our memory and cognition, while it improves our focus and our performance in the face of challenge. This is why it's best to think of stress as a *frenemy*; it's both good for us *and* bad for us, something that becomes obvious when we look at the inverse-U curve of stress and benefit.

On the face of it, the stress response sounds like a simple, binary teeter-totter: you're either in fight-flight or rest-digest. When we turn one off, we turn the other one on. But in the living animal, the body's response to stress follows a classic bell curve of rising benefit, a tipping point and diminishing returns. If we're going to be good autonomic athletes, it's essential that we understand how the curve works and what it means in daily life.

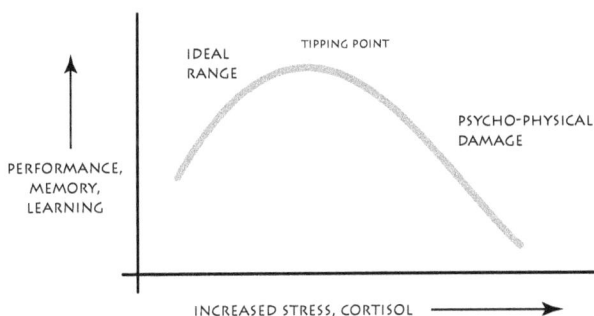

To begin, imagine a boring Sunday afternoon with nothing to do. You're camped out on the left side of the stress curve, nothing much is happening and you're bored. The relaxation might well feel good for a few hours, but from a performance standpoint, you're really not operating at a high level; your body and your brain are just idling.

Now suppose that you engage with some sort of challenge, marked by a certain degree of effort, ambiguity and risk. At this point, everything changes as rising levels of stress hormones drive powerful changes for the body, brain, and cognition. Metabolic fuels are released into the bloodstream to feed our attentive brains, stimulating the growth of new nerve cells, dendrites, and synapses. In this sweet spot, memory is sharp, and attention is focused.

This condition is sometimes described as *eustress*.

As stress increases, benefits also increase, but beyond the tipping point, the effect reverses itself and stress becomes destructive. Our cognitive, psychological, and spiritual resources begin to drain away, and our bodies are slower to recuperate from exertion, injury, and illness. In turn, this makes us increasingly vulnerable to other stressors, even those we would normally weather without a second thought. Aches and pains seem worse than normal, and we begin to worry about the trajectory of our health.

Over time, chronic activation of the stress response inhibits the growth and connectivity of precious neurons and can even damage brain centers that are involved in learning, memory, and impulse control. Key neurotransmitters such as dopamine become depleted, which leads to a loss of pleasure. If stress continues, our mood becomes increasingly serious, then grim. Our sense of humor declines, then disappears entirely. We stop laughing; we stop loving life.

At this point, we enter the dark world of disease, dysfunction, and depression. Stress hormones may even become neurotoxic, endangering neurons and even killing them outright. Chronic exposure erodes the structure and function of the hippocampus, a crucial brain center involved in explicit, short-term memory and learning. At this level, stress hormones become psychotoxic, leading to impulse control problems and substance abuse. We fall into a state of learned helplessness and begin to generalize our lack of control to other circumstances, even to those cases when control is in fact possible.

All of which sounds positively awful, but don't be overly alarmed. The brain also has a powerful ability to rebuild circuitry and structures that are damaged by stress and in fact, this is an utterly normal, routine process, a waxing and waning of synaptic arbors that shrink and expand under the rhythmic, daily influence of stress and stress hormones. In other words, it's normal to suffer some loss of connectivity as we push ourselves outside our comfort zones, and it's just as normal for the brain to rebuild degraded connections, especially during rest and sleep.

HEED THE WARNING SIGNS

The inverse-U curve provides some powerful life lessons that can inform our work, our health, and our activism. In the first place, it teaches us that stress has real value. In moderation, it's essential for learning, performance, and a good life. So instead of trying to make our lives stress free, the superior strategy is to seek an optimal level of challenge: the right kind of stress, in the right intensity, for the right duration. In other words, look for precision, not eradication. Whenever possible, fine-tune your adversities and your level of engagement.

The essential practice is to recognize the point of diminishing returns. As stress increases and you approach the tipping point, be alert for these warning signs:

- Anhedonia (loss of pleasure)

- Neophobia (avoidance of new things)

- Perseveration (mindless repetition of established habit patterns)

- Reduced ambiguity tolerance, increased extremism and black-and–white thinking

- Social withdrawal and isolation

- Cognitive distortions, especially overgeneralizing and short-term thinking

- Physical lethargy, poor sleep quality, decreased resilience

- Irritability; "making mountains out of molehills"

- Catastrophizing; worst-case thinking

- Decreased sense of humor and play

- Poor concentration and attention span

- Impulsive behaviors, reduced self-control

- Decision resistance, procrastination and impatience.

All of which makes us wonder about where we stand, not just as individuals, but as a culture at large. Are we coasting along on the left side of the curve, in the sweet spot of eustress, are we teetering on the tipping point of reversal, or are we headed towards the pain, dysfunction and disease of the right side?

Judging from modern mental health challenges and the widespread dysfunctional behavior we see in today's world, it's safe to say that we're in real danger. Many of us—even most of us—are marinating in cortisol, perilously close to the edge of disaster. And thus the challenge of our age: dampen the stress, reduce the fear, ease the pressure and shift our lives back to the left side of the curve. To put it another way, decreasing fear ought to be an explicit social focus, even a cultural and policy priority. To put it bluntly, most of us need to calm down.

WHAT'S DANGEROUS?

As we've seen, one of the crucial fundamentals of effective living—both in prehistory and the modern world—is to have an accurate understanding of what's dangerous and what isn't. In other words, the challenge is to be afraid of the right things, in the right degree, at the right time. It's a waste of autonomic energy to turn on your stress response early, late, or worst of all, over things that aren't really dangerous in the first place. The fundamental challenge is to be wary of real tigers, while letting go of those that only appear real.

Naturally, all of us struggle with this kind of judgment call and the experience is surely a human universal. We all get worked up over perceived or imaginary threats, only to realize days or weeks later that things weren't nearly as bad as we'd feared. Mark Twain understood this clearly: "I've had a lot of worries in my life, most of which never happened." As we get older, we come to recognize this tendency with greater clarity; something bugs us and we feel the inclination to react, but experience tells us that it's probably not as bad as we think.

All of which makes good neurological and evolutionary sense. That is, the fight-flight system is hyper-sensitive and armed with a hair trigger; it's really easy to turn on, but it takes some time in the right conditions to turn off. This might seem oddly asymmetrical, but given our history, it could hardly be otherwise. After all, life on the open grasslands of East Africa was no picnic; hungry predators were everywhere and any day could be your last.

In this kind of world, it paid to have a hair-trigger stress response. If that rustle in the bushes turns out to be an authentic threat, you're ready to fight or flee, but if it turns out to be a mouse, little harm is done. The consequence is that the average human is slightly paranoid and over-re-active, a tendency that becomes even more pronounced when we're chronically stressed. In other words, we're hair-trigger primates, loose in a highly challenging and ambiguous modern world.

This understanding is extremely valuable. Once we be-come aware of our hyper-active, hair-trigger tendencies, we're in a better position to let some things go. That thing in the bushes with the pointy ears probably isn't a tiger at all; we're just over-reacting. Likewise, we have a greater sense of tolerance and compassion for the hyper-active, hair-trigger people around us. They're not bad people; they're just wired for fast action in a prehistoric world.

In any case, it's essential that we learn to make distinc-tions between real and false tigers. A real tiger is a genuine threat to your life, your loved ones, or the life-supporting systems around you. This kind of threat demands decisive, immediate action or evasion; you've got to do something now. In contrast, a false tiger only appears dangerous. It triggers a stress response, but on closer examination, it proves to be harmless and can safely be ignored.

Likewise, it's crucial to make distinctions between slow and fast tigers. Naturally, we're programmed to respond most strongly to the fast tigers, the carnivores that are chasing us across the grassland. In contrast, slow tigers don't arouse much of our attention, even though the con-sequences might be far more consequential in the long run. This is obviously the case with our ecological crisis. Decades ago, it may have been a slow tiger, but now it's accelerating with terrifying speed and is about to become ferociously dangerous.

Unfortunately, impulsive humans are notoriously bad at sorting out real and false tigers, especially when we're under stress, and especially when living in a modern world full of ambiguous threats. This suggests a reality-based approach and a scientific orientation. Science, as it turns out, is quite adept at identifying dangerous beasts and in turn, helping us to adjust our responses.

But science can't tell us everything about what's dangerous and it can't tell us much about how to sort out the tigers in our personal lives either. Is my annoying, dysfunctional neighbor a genuine threat to my life? Maybe. What about the chaos in my workplace, the traffic on the highway, the incomprehensible medical bill on my desk, or the rising dominance of an opposing political party? Are these real tigers, or just noise in the modern system?

There can be no ultimate answers here, but on a personal level, simply asking the question makes an enormous difference in the quality and trajectory of our lives. The very act of inquiry gives us a chance to react more appropriately. So slow down, take a breath and ask yourself about the true nature of what you're facing. If you can let go of the false carnivores in your life, you'll have more energy left for dealing with the real ones.

YIN AND YANG...

But what's to be done when we do find ourselves mired in stress, anxiety, and overwhelm? There are dozens of practices available, but to simplify, there are really just two basic strategies. On one hand, we have what we might call the "yang" arts, the various practices that help us increase control over our circumstances; we manipulate the world with our hands, tools, and knowledge, and in the process, come to feel better about things in general. On the other hand are the "yin" practices in which we relinquish control, accepting and yielding to our circumstances without resistance. What makes this duality fascinating is that both approaches can work and as it turns out, being ambidextrous might well be the best approach.

The yang arts begin with the recognition that all animals need a sense of power and control to thrive. When nonhuman animals are placed in laboratory conditions that decrease their sense of control, they show biological markers of stress, but when control is restored, they do better. In a typical example, a rodent that can turn off an electric shock does better than a rodent that can't, even when the levels of electrical stress are precisely the same. Predictability helps too—a rat that gets a warning light before an electric shock does better than one that gets no such warning, even when the levels of stress are identical.

In this sense, the obvious solution to stress lies in focusing our attention on executing our work and regaining control. When our lives are in chaos, we need to accomplish vital tasks that will help us get a grip on our situation; we've got to redouble our efforts and get the work done.

There's no real mystery here. The yang arts are all about task management and the fundamentals of modern living: planning our days and weeks, using a calendar, budgeting our time, making to-do lists, and keeping our schedules in order. Do the planning, get the work done, gain a sense of control, and in turn, your stress will diminish. To put it simply, work works.

Education also increases our sense of power and control, especially when it's relevant to actual circumstances on the ground. Practical knowledge gives us options, and in turn, makes the world seem less arbitrary and more predictable. Even physical strength training can give us a feeling of mastery and resilience. When we work our bodies against gravity and build our physical competence, the rest of world begins to feel more manageable by comparison.

Power and control are essential antidotes to stress, but they can only take us so far. After all, there are only so many situations in the world that the human animal can control. Even with the most advanced tools, technologies, and knowledge, there are very real limits to what we can do. And when it comes to the hyper-complex, non-linear realities of people, social relationships, culture and modern large-scale systems, our best efforts are likely to be limited. If we persist in our efforts to control the uncontrollable, we not only stress ourselves unnecessarily, we also wreak havoc with the people and systems around us.

This is precisely why the yin arts of letting go are so important. This approach, sometimes described as "reversed effort," is a deliberate releasing of whatever it is that's bugging us. In this art, we take care of ourselves as need be with the yang arts, then we relinquish and relax. This approach is particularly useful in dealing with the irritating and annoying false tigers that are so widespread in the modern world: spam calls, tailgaters on the highway, noise makers. If it's a false tiger, let it go. Save your energy for the real predators.

In contrast to the yang arts, yin strategies are humble in nature. We bow before the big forces of nature. We bow before the hyper-complex, non-linear realities of bodies, ecosystems, social systems and the biosphere herself. We relinquish attachment to any particular outcome. We accept our powerlessness in the face ambiguity and uncertainty. We acknowledge our ignorance.

On the face of it, this "let it be" approach may well seem easy enough, but raised in a thoroughly yang culture as we are, it may well feel alien, even absurd. Raised from birth to take charge and "just do it," the whole idea of leaving things alone might well seem weak and nonsensical. But exercising the yin doesn't mean simply giving up in the face of adversity or living on our knees. It means picking our battles. It means being powerful at the right time and place. It means being fluid and adaptable. When we relinquish the desire for control, the autonomic nervous system relaxes and shifts away from fight-flight urgency. In the process, we regain our equanimity.

And so the obvious question: When to seek control and when to relinquish? When to yin and when to yang? Naturally, this reminds us of the Serenity Prayer, written by American theologian Reinhold Niebuhr:

> God, grant me the serenity to accept the things I cannot change, the courage to change the things I can, and wisdom to know the difference.

Well said, but then again, not really much help. After all, who really knows the difference? It's always a judgment call and all of us, even the most intelligent and level-headed among us have gotten it backwards on occasion. Are we to exercise serenity in accepting threats like climate chaos and the biodiversity crisis, things so enormous that personal efforts seem insignificant? Or should we fight on principle, even against overwhelming odds, because to do otherwise would be unacceptable? Maybe it's not enough to simply "change the things we can." Maybe we should fight long and hard, even in the face of overwhelming odds.

In any case, one thing seems certain: every human animal, every aspiring artist and activist must become fluent in both yin and yang strategies. One-trick ponies are destined to fail in a hyper-complex, dynamic world. If all you've got are the yang arts of power and control, you'll inevitably destroy your world and create more stress for everyone. If all you've got are the yin arts of acceptance and yielding, you'll get run over, abused, violated, and be of no use to anyone.

The solution: know them both, practice them both. Whatever it is you're doing, reserve the capability to do the other.

BEAUTY AND BEASTS

As we've seen, the autonomic nervous system is capped by a sophisticated set of brain structures that interpret reality and drive the autonomic in one direction or the other. Our brains are constantly assigning meaning to the conditions around us, translating reality into feelings of safety or danger.

So naturally, attention is a vital part of the process. If we pay lots of attention to danger, hostility and the unfriendliness of the world, we keep ourselves locked into a state of emergency activation, which ultimately compromises our health and performance. If we pay more attention to the friendly aspects of the world, our bodies simply work better. This is why many teachers advise us to pay attention to what we're paying attention to; a skill that some call meta-cognition.

Ideally, we'd pay attention to the world without prejudice, watching for dangerous tigers *and* beautiful sunsets. We'd be flexible and ambidextrous in our focus, allowing both the friendliness and unfriendliness of the world to co-exist in our consciousness. But depending on our history and personality, most of us are inclined to fall back onto one attentional style or the other.

Some of us prefer to attend exclusively to the friendliness of the world. Just ignore the nasty things; the glass is always half-full and everything is going to be OK. This is great practice for keeping ourselves in a healing state of rest-digest or feed-and-breed, which in turn is good for our long term health, but in the extreme, it becomes problematic. If all we ever look for are rainbows and butterflies, our lives become increasingly irrelevant, isolated, and ultimately meaningless.

On the other hand, it's easy to fall into the habit of looking exclusively at the unfriendly elements of our world; the dangerous, toxic, and hostile beasts that prowl the perimeters of our camps. In fact, there are so many ferocious carnivores in the mix these days, it's hard not to see them everywhere we look. This kind of attention can give us a high level of relevance and short-term functionality, but it's ultimately corrosive to our health, our disposition, and eventually, our effectiveness.

As always, the dose makes the poison and the sweet spot must lie somewhere in the center. This is why the activist would do well to balance her attention between friend-liness and unfriendliness, between danger and comfort, between threat and safety. Think of the practice this way: For every terrifying future-hostile carnivore you encounter, try to see at least one nurturing aspect of the world around you. For every act of deforestation or habitat destruction, look for a flock of birds, a running stream, or an alpine meadow. For every new fossil fuel project or pipeline that's approved, enjoy the comfort of the people closest to you. For every atrocity committed against land and people, find at least one reminder of the beauty of what we're trying to save.

TREAT PEOPLE LIKE ANIMALS

In the standard narrative of stress management, the vast majority of advice is pointed directly at individuals who want to feel better. We're feeling anxious and overwhelmed and experts are quick to step up and help us get back to a state of equanimity. What's lost in this conversation is how our understanding of stress can help inform our interactions with one another, especially our activism and our martial artistry. And we start by learning to treat people like animals.

This is no joke. Yes, it's fun to declare that the people around you are "going wild" or that getting people to do things is "like herding cats." And we've all used the phrase "they treated us like animals" when suffering some sort of abusive treatment. But this is a serious piece of advice, one that can make us far more effective in our relationships and our efforts to create change.

To begin, there simply can be no denying the biological

nature of our bodies. As children of evolution, every detail of our anatomy, physiology and behavior can be traced back to the multi-million year history of our hominid line. Every system in our brains and bodies has a precursor and an ancestry and nearly all of it is shared with other creatures. In actual fact, our bodies are not arbitrary and neither is our behavior. Like it or not, recognize it or not, we are kin with the rest of the living world.

So how do we work with the human animals around us? The good news is that the fundamentals are well understood. Writing in Scientific American (December 2005) professor Robert Sapolsky offered a concise explanation and a road map for working with stressed-out human animals. As he put it,

> Individuals are more likely to activate a stress response and are more at risk for a stress sensitive disease if they...
>
> • feel as if they have minimal control
>
> • feel as if they have no predictive information
>
> • have few outlets for their frustration
>
> • lack social support

In effect, Sapolsky has given us a framework for working with our friends, families, employees, allies, and maybe even our adversaries. Whenever possible, give people more control, better predictive information, and make sure they have outlets (hobbies, sports, or any kind of activity outside the stress domain) And above all, make sure that they have some sort of humane, authentic, and meaningful social support.

In this process, it's essential that your people "feel felt." No matter our background, history, or culture, all of us have a deep-seated desire to be recognized; to feel seen, heard, felt, understood, and respected. This is a human universal; people of every age, culture, origin, and status crave this experience. Even the Na'vi, the fictional indigenous people of Pandora depicted in the movie Avatar, address one another with the honorific "I see you."

This social need is far more than a superficial emotional desire. It's rock-solid biology that goes all the way to the deepest levels of our bodies and our nervous systems, as real as our need for food and water. When the human animal feels recognized and appreciated, the world just feels safer and in turn, the autonomic nervous system goes into action, repairing tissues and opening up the aperture of cognition and creativity. Without question, the experience of being recognized is a powerful and inexpensive form of medicine in its own right.

All of which may well seem obvious, but on the other hand, "feeling felt" is in real danger of disappearing in the modern world; we might even call it an endangered human experience. As society becomes ever more automated and transactional, the human animal often gets left in the dust. Profit, productivity, objectives, goals, and above all, efficiency—all are extremely destructive to our deepest social needs. As we drive relentlessly towards the bottom line, we leapfrog over essential human experiences and in the process, create a society of increasing alienation. Is it any wonder that we see an epidemic of loneliness in the modern world? When human relationships are squeezed into sterile, automated transactions, there's not much left for the human animal to live for.

For the martial artist, this suggests some solid strategies for action. First, it's safe to assume that most people you meet—both allies and adversaries—are starving for social recognition; a great many people in the modern world simply don't feel felt. And deprived of this basic need, they're going to be on edge, stressed, erratic, depressed, or otherwise dysfunctional. In other words, the strange behavior of the people around you might simply be down to the fact that they aren't feeling recognized or appreciated. Of course they're going off the rails. You would too.

This understanding moves us towards greater patience, compassion and the realization that our adversaries might not be the monsters they appear to be. Maybe they just need someone to listen to them on occasion. Maybe they just need to get off the transactional, for-profit treadmill and have some authentic human encounters for a change. And just maybe, we can give them what they need. So listen to your people and make sure they feel felt. Slow down and pay attention. If your opponent begins to feel recognized, he might just give up his resistance altogether. It's definitely worth a shot.

STRESS AND CHARACTER

As we've seen, stress is a frenemy with both positive and negative effects on our bodies and our lives. But there's a hidden upside that we rarely hear about in the standard narrative. That is, stress can have a powerfully revealing effect on our lives, our personalities, and our character. In short, stress can tell us who we are.

Think of your life as an activist, artivist, or martial artist. As you engage with the world and focus your efforts against entrenched power, you're going to experience friction, frustration, and exhaustion. Defeats are common and it's easy to fall into the quagmire of resignation, learned helplessness and despair. All of which sounds like another round of bad news, but we can find some surprising inspiration in an unlikely source: the screenwriters of Hollywood.

Think of a typical movie. No matter the genre, the action usually begins with a setting, a protagonist, and an inciting incident—a stressor of some kind. There's something amiss in the world: a challenge, a problem, a mystery, an injury or an illness. Normal conditions are thrown out of order; something is broken, something doesn't add up. The audience wonders: How will the protagonist respond? In particular, what is her character? What is she made of? Will she stand up to the challenge with courage and resolve or will she buckle under the pressure?

This is where the screenwriter goes to work, escalating the stress on the protagonist over the course of the movie. The inciting incident is challenge enough, but now there's an additional stressor, then another, always ratcheting up the pressure until finally, stress reaches a climax and the character of the protagonist is revealed, for better or for worse. She either rises to the challenge or folds and goes down in defeat.

This is a tried-and-true formula for modern cinema and makes for solid entertainment, but it also holds a powerful life lesson for all of us. As stress escalates, it threatens to grind us down and wear us out, but it also provides powerful illumination into our character. In short, it tells us who we are and what we're made of. In this way, the stress of activism is a priceless form of education.

The beauty of this perspective is that it helps us reframe our experience. As stress closes in, it's easy to get wrapped up in the nastiness of the whole thing. But if we can step back and let the experience teach us, we'll find out who we really are. And just maybe, you're doing better than you think.

PRACTICES

Once you start treating yourself and relating
to the world as an empowered human
being instead of a hapless consumer drone,
something remarkable happens. Your cynicism
dissolves. Your instincts sharpen.

Kalle Lasn
Manifesto for World Revolution

So here we are, trying to make a go of it as activists, artivists, and on some days, simply as functional human beings. But our predicament is relentless and there's a good chance that you've got one foot in the mental health quagmire already. In all likelihood, you're suffering from one or more of the common afflictions of our era: anxiety, depression, attention disorders and all the rest. You might even feel like there's something fundamentally wrong with you.

All of which makes an odd sort of sense. After all, the standard health and wellness narrative tells us that these conditions are simply afflictions of the individual. Your body is nothing more than a stand-alone, isolated mechanism with faulty parts. There's something wrong with your nervous system, your brain, your neurotransmitter levels, or most problematic of all, your psychological disposition and your relationship with the world. Your health—for better and for worse—has almost nothing to do with the world or the social systems you inhabit. It's all about you.

But this kind of "reasoning" is a flawed conceptual hangover from the early days of the scientific revolution, when clocks and mechanisms were held as ideal models for animal bodies, life on earth and even the cosmos as a whole. And in this paradigm, it made a certain kind of sense to view people as isolated, individual units, subject to various malfunctions, illnesses and injuries. Just put the body on a laboratory bench, start probing, and you'll eventually get to the root of the problem. Ultimately, the body is just another thing, a medical object.

But today we know better, or to put it more accurately, we *should* know better. Scientific advances of the last century, coupled with the knowledge of native and indigenous peoples, shows us clearly that human bodies are deeply embedded—even continuous—with the world. We are not and never have been stand-alone organisms. The state of our bodies, minds and spirits is constantly being sculpted by physical, social, historical and biological processes that lie outside our skin. In other words, when it comes to the state of our bodies, big systems matter; the world matters, context and circumstance matter. In turn, this realization puts our experience in a new light. As a deeply embedded animal, your suffering is almost certainly a reflection of the conditions that you're living in.

To put it another way, you are almost certainly *not* diseased. If biology and big history teach us anything, it's that modern humans are living in radically altered, unnatural circumstances; it's no exaggeration to say that we are living in an alien environment.

With this in mind, just imagine this scenario: Put your dog in the garage—an alien environment for any large mammal—and leave him there for weeks and months on end. Feed him on schedule but allow no interactions with people, other dogs, toys, or the natural world.

After a time, your dog is certain to develop a variety of psycho-physical afflictions. His coat will look dull and dingy, he'll be chewing on everything in sight, and he'll be neurotic as hell. You can bring in a veterinarian in to treat these afflictions individually, but how much sense does that make? That's because, in a very real sense, there's nothing wrong with your dog. His body is simply responding the way any animal would respond to severe incarceration in an unnatural environment.

The same goes for other mammals, including humans. Physician and trauma specialist Gabor Mate encourages us to see modern psycho-physical illness "not as a cruel twist of fate or some nefarious mystery but rather as an *expected and therefore normal consequence of abnormal, unnatural circumstances.*" In other words, you are that dog.

For some, this view might feel odd and unsettling, but it's actually quite liberating. That's because, in all likelihood, your depression, insomnia, disordered attention, and anxiety are not your fault. You may feel terrible, but in a biological sense, your condition is utterly normal. The problem isn't you; it's the garage you're living in.

This insight gives us permission to move forward as individuals and as activists. To be sure, you may still feel the pull of the quagmire, but now you can turn your attention outward, to the systems that have created the abnormal living conditions in the first place. At this point, your activism becomes medicinal, for you and for the people around you.

Getting out of the garage of the modern world would be an ideal move for today's human animal, but most of us are severely limited in what's possible. We'd like to move and live somewhere that is ecologically and socially humane, somewhere that's more consistent with our evolutionary origins, but without some windfall affluence, such a thing is almost impossible. Even for people with windfall affluence, high-end living isn't really what the human animal needs anyway. It's merely a fancy, upgraded version of the garage, complete with granite counter tops.

Nevertheless, there are things that we can do, things that we really must do to maintain our equilibrium and health in the face of today's extreme circumstances. These are the practices, essential supporting behaviors for successful activism. If we're to have any chance of success in taking on the ecological crisis of today's world, we've got to do this work. And remember, in a world that seems hell-bent on strip mining our bodies and our lives in the naked pursuit of profit, taking care of yourself is a revolutionary act.

THE FUNDAMENTALS

Of course, we've all heard the basics by now. Almost everyone in the modern world has heard about the importance of regular movement (exercise), real food enjoyed with family and friends, good sleep, meaningful work, and lots of rest. There's not much left to be said about the details.

But there *is* a great deal to be said about context and meaning of these practices. Unfortunately, the standard health and wellness narrative leads us astray right at the outset, where the practices are pitched squarely at the individual. In fact, the whole point of the enterprise is to enhance personal health, appearance, and performance. And so the common refrain: "I'm practicing yoga, running, cycling and so on so that I can live *my* best life, avoid illness, and live a long time."

This is the answer sold to us through thousands of lifestyle and wellness publications. Health is for you, or me, but never has anything to do with us. In essence, the purpose of the practices is to create personal health islands that will keep us safe and happy. Once we've done our sets, reps, and mileage, we can safely ignore the rest of the world, content and comfortable in our well-sculpted, perfectly conditioned bodily bunkers.

Even worse, the practices are heavily focused on destinations, which is to say, the emphasis is on the rewards that we'll enjoy after we endure a long and unpleasant exercise and diet journey. As with so many incentive programs in the modern world, the practices are pitched as "do this and you'll get that." Just keep grinding out the sets, reps, and mileage and one day you'll be fit and happy. If you suffer long enough and hard enough, you'll get to enjoy a health payoff at the end. All of which sets us up for failure. Who wants to suffer for a reward in some distant future? Most of us would rather head for the pub.

So yes, the practices are good for us as individuals and yes, we might well enjoy some health rewards down the line, but if we're going to live a life of relevance, we need to reframe the entire experience as something more expansive and meaningful. In this, the ultimate purpose of health is not to hoard it or possess it, but to give it away, to return our vital energy to the social and natural world that gave us life in the first place. This gives us a broader, more meaningful sense of what we're doing and why we're doing it.

To put it another way, the point of the practices is to reweave our lives back into the flow of the natural world. Obviously, we all want to feel good and look good, but in this view, the shape of your body doesn't much matter. Your athletic performance doesn't matter, and neither does your longevity. And in a limited, bio-medical sense, even your health itself doesn't really matter. What does matter is your ability to carry the fight forward, to work for the world, to show up even in the face of overwhelming opposition and stress. If you're going to be an effective eco-warrior or artivist, you've got to do the practices that keep you strong.

With that in mind, try dedicating your next workout to the natural world. Dedicate your weight-lifting session to the forest, your cardio to the atmosphere, your meditation to the ocean, your yoga session to future generations, your therapeutic rest to the planet itself. You won't win any races or medals with this kind of approach and your friends will almost certainly call you crazy, but it's good, meaningful work nonetheless.

FOOD

The first practice is all about food. We all like to eat and most of us have opinions about what constitutes a balanced diet. We're surrounded by mountains of nutritional information, but we're also bedeviled be anxiety over the whole process. There are supposedly "good foods" and "bad foods," and new food-like products appear in the stores every day. We try to do our homework, but even the experts disagree on key issues. Just try getting a straight answer to "How much protein do I need?" or even "How much water should I drink?" We can be sure that our ancestors never had so much unease about what to eat each day.

Unfortunately, the standard narratives around food include several highly problematic ideas and assumptions. The first is what Michael Pollan and others have described as *nutritionism*, the focus on single ingredients or elements that are claimed to have special powers. Ever since the discovery of Vitamin C and its healing effect on scurvy, nutritional science has gone all in on this reductionistic approach. Along the way, we've broken our food into pieces and in the process, lost contact with its original power and meanings.

Nutritionism tells us that "This ingredient is good for this medical condition, this one is good before a workout, this one is good for recovery, this one is good for gaining weight, this one is good for losing weight." And so on. And with thousands of nutritional elements and millions of possible combinations, there's simply no way for the average eater to track it all; which is precisely why so many of us simply give up and revert to whatever happens to taste good, especially the ultra-processed food-like substances that surround us.

Closely related is the popular "food-is-fuel" metaphor. According to this narrative, our bodies are nothing more than fancy vehicles and food is nothing more than "gas in the tank." Obviously, this is a doubly problematic metaphor. Not only does it strip our food of all meaning beyond biochemistry, it also likens our food to a fossil-fuel extract. In other words, having a meal is just like pulling into the gas station.

All of which is plenty disturbing on its own, but the even bigger issue has to do with origin stories or more accurately, the *lack* of origin stories. That is, our food is now presented to us out of thin air. In grocery stores and restaurants across the modern world, there it is. Rarely do we hear the back story of where our food comes from, how it was produced, or who was involved. It simply appears as if by magic, brought to us by invisible processes, with invisible people doing invisible work, all so we can eat with the maximum possible convenience.

Paradoxically, we're victims of our agricultural and industrial success. Modern farmers and producers have been so effective in bringing vast quantities of food into our lives that it's all taken for granted and for affluent people in the modern world, food is almost free. Always handy, always available, we hardly give it a second thought. For most consumers, there's no need to worry about habitat destruction, depletion of biodiversity, or the horrific conditions that both human and non-human animals have to endure in the process. In a sense, we're eating food without a history, food without a story. If we truly understood the ecological and moral damage that comes with industrial food production, we'd lose our appetites in a hurry.

It hardly needs to be said that his condition is wickedly abnormal. For the vast majority of our history as humans, no one ever talked about macronutrients, micronutrients, food-as-fuel, food-as-reward, or food-as-fun. Food always had intrinsic meaning that connected people directly to one another and to habitat. Everyone in your tribe would have known the back story of almost every meal. Every bite came with an account of someone's hunting or gathering and in the process, food served as a bond between humans and habitat, between people and one another.

So what's the practice? Obviously, we'd all be better off if everyone grew their food in community gardens and took the time to understand and appreciate the back stories of what we're eating. But for most of us, most of the time, we're forced to participate in a toxic system to some degree.

Nevertheless, we are not powerless. Remember, you're not just throwing down carbs, protein, and fat, you're eating a story, participating in a narrative of your people's relationship to habitat and one another. With this realization, we shift our attention to the meanings that come with every meal. Don't get distracted by the plasticized front stories that circulate across modern media; focus on the back stories of your food and keep it in awareness. Then, enjoy your food as our ancestors did; strengthening the bond with habitat and one another. It's not a perfect solution, but it's a start.

And naturally, all this reminds us of Michael Pollan's legendary advice about healthy eating: "Eat real food. Not too much. Mostly plants." To which we might well add one more quip: "Eat real food. Not too much. Mostly plants. And remember the back story of what you're eating."

MOVEMENT

In conventional prescriptions for self-care, we're usually counseled to "get some exercise" and it's generally offered as a magic bullet that will cure nearly everything that ails us. This is actually close to being true, but once again, the standard prescription gets us off on the wrong foot. That's because "exercise" is actually a modern invention and strictly speaking, isn't even part of the original, historically-normal human repertoire.

In fact, exercise is a product of the modern industrial revolution, something we can tell just by looking: gyms that look suspiciously like factories, with treadmills and machines in perfect rows, people tracking every set and rep with digital devices. But this is profoundly abnormal. Prior to the industrial age, people got plenty of physical movement in the course of their daily lives. First hunting and gathering, walking and occasionally running, then dance, agriculture, and craft. For the vast majority of our history, we've been moving our bodies, entirely without the help of gyms, machines, amplified music or personal trainers.

The same holds true for non-human animals. We never observe other primates doing anything resembling exercise. They hunt, gather, eat, mate, play, fight and flee, but never do they perform repetitive movements for the sake of "staying in shape." They move their bodies for pleasure, to play, explore, or stay alive, but otherwise, they eat or rest.

This suggests a broader view and a new appreciation for context. When we exercise, we engage in a narrow physical specialization, but when practice natural movement, we put ourselves back into community with every mammal that's ever lived, a deep heritage that goes back more than a hundred million years. In the process, we celebrate our kinship with the natural world and make ourselves part of something much, much larger than ourselves.

In the process, we benefit in surprising ways. In conventional conversations about movement (aka exercise), advocates are quick to list the medical and physiological benefits: decreased blood pressure, improved blood chemistry, increased metabolism, stronger muscles and improved brain function. These advantages are very real, but even better, physical movement has profound psychological benefits in the way it increases our sense of control in the world. This can be a powerful antidote to the sense of powerless that so many of us feel in today's world.

It's easy to imagine how this works. Choose an exercise of any type and think about how it feels, not just in your limbs, but in the totality of your experience. Strength training is the most obvious example: the very act of lifting something heavy gives us the feeling that we are competent, even powerful actors in the world; we are taking control of our situation and our lives. Other types of vigorous movement have a similar effect, but no matter the form, it's all about developing our sense of agency and effectiveness. This is a vital experience for modern living and sustainable activism.

HAVE A MOVEMENT SNACK

In the standard view, we're accustomed to talking about exercise as something that's performed at particular times as "a workout," but this too is a rather abnormal idea; we simply cannot imagine our hunting and gathering ancestors doing anything like it. Why should our physicality be concentrated in a single burst, in a single place, at a particular time of day?

A better idea is to distribute our movement throughout the day in periodic "movement snacks." The idea here is to keep updating our connection with the body, keep refreshing our sense of physicality and control. These mini sessions provide an essential break from our digital work and can reverse the effects of cognitive overload, chronic postural flexion and the sedentary blues.

All you need is a small open area, and maybe a medicine ball if you've got one. A few minutes of arm swings, squats and lunges will bring your body-mind back into integration. You'll get your breathing turned on and get your metabolism up and running. For best results, repeat often and don't sweat over what your co-workers might happen to think.

Ultimately, the idea here is not to get in shape, maximize your fitness, athletic performance, or body beautiful. Rather, the point is to feel your animal vitality, your intrinsic resilience, and your physical capability. In the process, you'll re-establish the mind-body unity that's been disrupted by the acute or chronic stress experience of our modern, alien environment. It doesn't matter how many calories you're burning or what your heart rate happens to be. It doesn't matter what kind of shoes you're wearing, how fast you're going, how much you're lifting or what your electronic device has to say about it all. What matters is how you *feel*. If you can feel the signal of a strong, vigorous animal body in action, you're doing it right.

BREATH

When it comes to practices for buffering the negative effects of stress, most of us have heard about the importance of working with the breath. Advocates claim that the practice has almost magical properties that will do wonders for our state of mind and body. We've heard it a thousand times.

But just as commonly, we also tend to ignore the advice. The breath is one of the most familiar aspects of our experience so it's easy to ignore. We've been breathing since the very beginning, so it's hard to imagine that it's special in any way. Surely there must be something else out there, something exotic or specialized that will give us the relief that we're seeking. Why bother with something so unremarkable?

Not only is the breath hyper-familiar, it also seems relatively weak. We try the practice once or twice and nothing dramatic happens. Maybe we experience some momentary relief, but in comparison to the crushing stress burden we're experiencing, it seems like nothing at all. We want dramatic solutions and we want them now.

But little things can be extremely powerful, especially when practiced with diligence over the course of months and years. With repetition, our breath practice translates into substantive changes to body, spirit, and disposition. And in fact, it's deceptively powerful medicine.

Not only does the breath bring us life-giving oxygen, rhythmic contractions of the diaphragm massage our abdominal organs and in the process, send calming messages to the brain via the vagus nerve. Even better, a strong set of breathing muscles can support our biomechanics by increasing intra-abdominal pressure when squatting and lifting. All of which is supportive of our spines and low backs.

But the breath is far more than a tonic for our stressed-out and disintegrated physiology. It's also a cure for our distraction and amnesia, a return to the core truth of our experience as human animals. The breath is home, or to put it another way, working with the breath is like going back in time, back to a time before language, before distraction, before the insanity of the modern world.

So how do we practice? We've all heard advice about the importance of "belly breathing" and "diaphragmatic breathing," but there's really no single technique that we need to master; the body really does know what to do. In fact, the human animal is no different than any other mammal, which is to say, we're wired for effective, life-supporting breath. Barring some catastrophic trauma or the intense pressure of the modern age, all of us are fully capable of making it work. We're smart enough to take long, deep breaths when we're flustered or overcome with complexity. All we really need to do is more of what we already know how to do.

That said, some practices are particularly beneficial:

Belly breathing; the more the better.

Long slow exhales; the more the better.

Over-breathing: intentional exaggeration of what's already happening. Powerful inhales followed by total relaxation.

Whole body breathing: every cell participates in the expansion and relaxation.

Extended breathing, particularly on the inhale. Imagine your skin as permeable and it absorbs the totality of your surroundings—the life in your neighborhood, your region, your planet. Feel the continuity between your body and the life around you. On the exhale, feel the entire world relaxing.

Creative breathing: imagine vast, swirling, expansive clouds on the inhale or powerful ocean waves that move your entire experience with each breath.

Another vital element is to direct your attention to your lower abdomen and a point that Chinese call the *dantian*, or *tan tien*. This is a vital center for the movement of *chi* or life energy that flows through the body. There's plenty of history, sophistication, and outright mysticism surrounding the dantian, but for our purposes, we can think of it as a focal point for breathing and physical movement. As you breathe, think 3-dimensionally; your focus should be a bit below the navel, deep in the center of your torso. Keep your attention here as your diaphragm does its magic.

No matter which particular practice feels right for you, keep paying attention and become a connoisseur of your experience. When in doubt, when distressed, go back to your center. When angry, when depressed, when confused, when fatigued, all are opportunities to pay attention to the vital rhythm.

And above all, practice rewiring your reactions to the events and stresses of the modern world. For every event that challenges your equanimity or triggers your sense of despair, return your attention to your breath. It's more powerful than it appears.

MEDITATION

In a moment of stopping, we break the spell between past result and automatic reaction. When we pause, we can notice the actual experience, the pain or pleasure, fear or excitement. In the stillness before our habits arise, we become free.

Jack Kornfield

Chaos, confusion, complexity—the lions and tigers and bears of our modern world are everywhere, especially for the activist. Every day serves up another avalanche of tasks, urgencies and responsibilities that must be attended to. We try to keep up with it all by multitasking, but most of us have gotten the memo from the neuroscience community by now. That is, the brain only attends to one thing at a time; when we attempt to manage multiple tasks simultaneously, the brain simply increases speed in switching from one point of attention to another. In moderation, we can manage it, but this rapid alternation of attention eventually takes a toll on our equanimity and even our health.

Overwhelmed by modern life and frustrated with conventional approaches, many of us turn to meditation for relief. Research suggests that regular practice reduces inflammation, lowers cortisol, and reduces anxiety, depression, anger, and fatigue. It also stimulates the vagus nerve, a powerful player in the autonomic nervous system that helps with healing, tissue repair, inflammation control, and psycho-physical rejuvenation.

The list of benefits is impressive, but once again, it's important to frame our discussion the right way. In our highly individualistic culture, meditation is often presented as yet another means of self-improvement, but this is likely to be a step in the wrong direction. In fact, the very act of trying to improve ourselves strengthens our sense of self, which in turn sets us up for more duality and in turn, conflict and anxiety. A better approach would be to think of meditation as a practice of non-self. We aren't trying to make ourselves better; we're trying to let go of our ego and merge ourselves with our bodies and the world. When we succeed, we experience less self, less duality, and in turn, less suffering.

In any case, meditation gives us a chance to step outside the complexity of our normal, daily lives and observe exactly what we're up to. In the process, it gives us an increased understanding of our experience. When we allow the chattering, judgmental mind to come to rest, we begin to actually feel what we're feeling. As we let go of the noise of the modern world, we begin to feel the life coursing through our bodies, via the breath.

From a mindbody point of view, meditation offers us vital experiential proof that we can coexist with ourselves. Sit quietly for a while and behold—nothing bad happens. Our minds might get distracted and we might waste some time ruminating on the dramas in our lives, but these things tend to fade away. In turn, it begins to dawn on us that it's not really necessary to spend every waking moment running away from ourselves or our predicaments. It's not necessary to surround ourselves with distraction and compulsive activity. It's okay to just be.

The experience is calming, but it's far more than even that. When we abandon our internal chatter and focus on our bodies and our breath, we might even feel a sense of reunification with the totality of life on Earth and the power that goes with it. When we relinquish our compulsive narration about our troubles, we're left with a direct experience of a body that's literally millions of years old and continuous with all life. This takes us out of our isolation and back into integration. In this sense, the medical benefits of meditation pale in comparison.

Unfortunately, meditation is often presented as a complex, daunting practice that takes decades to master. There are dozens of styles, hundreds of books, thousands of teachers, and according to some, layer upon layer of sophistication. This diversity makes for some interesting conversation, but it also distracts us from the essential simplicity of the experience.

In fact, there's no wrong way to do it. As one meditation teacher puts it, "Just sit down, shut up and pay attention." Turn off your phone and abandon your concerns about work, your to-do list, and all the things nagging at your mind. Forget about proper posture, breathing technique, attention, mindfulness, compassion, and loving kindness, at least for the moment. Keep it as simple as you can. As you relax, focus your attention on your breath, your most intimate ally, a safe and reliable friend that will show you the way to equanimity and calm.

In the process, it's helpful to recall some prompts commonly used by meditation teachers:

"Breathe with your whole body."

"Leave yourself alone."

"Trust your body."

"Feel what you're feeling."

"Imagine no effort."

And of course, "let it be."

Just sit quietly for a few minutes and pay attention.

Imagine yourself as being perfectly safe. Thoughts, images, and emotions will come, and some will be unwelcome, but don't resist. To put it another way, *don't try to change anything.* Your experience is never wrong, your animal body is never wrong, your mind is never wrong. Simply return your attention to your breath and feel what you're feeling.

As the Buddhist teacher Jack Kornfield put it, "Let go of the battle. Breathe quietly and let it be. Let your body relax and your heart soften. Open to whatever you experience without fighting." Accept what is happening, and before long your mind and body will relax. When this happens, you'll be ready to re-engage with clarity and creativity.

Of course, if you're anything like a normal human being, your attention will begin to wander almost immediately, and this is the moment of truth. If you try to strong-arm your attention back to your breath, you'll simply produce more duality and wind up even further away from your target. But passivity also fails. If you simply allow yourself to be swept up in whatever thoughts and imagery your mind cooks up, you'll never learn how to stabilize your attention. You'll simply have a nice daydreaming session.

The tricky part is that distraction feeds on itself. We drift off our focal point, each thought generates another association, memory, or image and before we know it, we're light years from our original intent. The solution, as the Buddhists point out, is compassion. There's nothing to be gained by abusing yourself for getting distracted. Every time you drift off target, you get another chance to practice.

So stick with it. When distraction intrudes on your experience, relax. Don't try to change anything. As Pema

Chodron, author of *When Things Fall Apart* advises, "soften and stay." Note the pain, the distraction and the emotion, then return to your breath. Observe the way your mind goes on journeys into the past and future. Observe the chatter, the commentary, and the random images that appear as if from nowhere. Then let it all go.

Whatever you do, keep it simple. In the popular imagination, many of us have come to believe that meditation is a path to some kind of higher, altered state of consciousness. Just as with almost everything else in the modern world, we want the special thing, the exceptional, the incredible, and the elite.

But we've got it entirely backwards. Meditation is not an altered, exceptional state; it's our normal state. It's our frenzied, anxious modern condition that's the altered state. When we meditate, we simply return to our historically normal condition of mind and body. So instead of reaching for something rare and astonishing, maybe we'd do better to reach for something modest. Don't worry about sophistication, advanced techniques, or mystical experiences. Stick with simplicity.

Of course, most of us claim to be too busy to bother with any of this. The practice takes time and produces no immediate payoff, so we simply avoid it in favor of more impulsive activity. But seen from another perspective, this makes no sense whatsoever. After all, we seem to have plenty of time for activities that bring noise, confusion, and complexity into our lives. Why not something that's proven to give us a sense of clarity, depth, and equanimity, if only for a few minutes each day? It's worth a try.

SLEEP

> Even a soul submerged in sleep is hard at work
> and helps make something of the world.
>
> Heraclitus

On first glance, it might seem odd that sleep would be listed as a "practice." After all, what could be easier and more natural? Just like any other mammal, we seek out slumber most nights and there seems to be nothing to it. For most of our history on Earth, sleep has been a simple pleasure, a mystery, and a fundamental part of life. In general, our ancestors went to sleep when they felt the need, and no one seemed to fret over the details.

Without question, sleep is an integral part of our animal heritage, something we ought to honor and respect. But in the modern world, human value is measured primarily by the ability to produce. People are considered worthy if they can get a lot done and in this environment, sleep is considered a nuisance and an adversary. We idolize people who claim to get by with less sleep, and in many circles, people who get enough sleep are considered slackers, a point of view voiced most notably by Thomas Edison, who declared sleep to be "a criminal waste of time."

To make matters worse, our modern environment is distinctly sleep-hostile. Our homes are often plagued by noise and light pollution, and hotels are commonly located next to freeways where rooms themselves are rarely dark or quiet. Even campgrounds in the mountains are no longer refuges for sleep; late arrivals and partiers keep the noise going until the small hours. It seems there's no place left that's truly dark, quiet, and safe to rest our heads.

Our problems with sleep began hundreds of years ago, with the advent of artificial light, a trend documented in detail by Paul Bogard in his book *The End of Night: Searching for Natural Darkness in an Age of Artificial Light*. By the end of the seventeenth century, many European cities had some form of artificial light and darkness has been under assault ever since. As Bogard tells it, we're now suffering from a very real darkness deficit. According to the World Atlas of Artificial Night Sky Brightness, two-thirds of the world's population no longer experiences a truly dark night and eight out of every ten children born today will never see the Milky Way. Most people are so awash in artificial light that their eyes never make a complete transition to night vision.

Not surprisingly, a substantial body of research concludes that people in the modern world are substantially sleep-deprived. In general, most of us go to bed too late and get up too early. A Gallup poll found that the average number of sleep hours per night dropped from almost 8 in 1942 to 6.8 in 2013. And as the world warms and nights become hotter, sleep is projected to become even shorter.

The consequences are no laughing matter: poor memory, poor judgment, decreased creativity, weight gain, muscle atrophy, suppressed immunity, and increased stress have all been linked to inadequate or poor-quality sleep. In 2005, the National Sleep Foundation found that 75 percent of American adults experienced sleep problems at least a few nights per week. According to Rubin Naiman at the Arizona Center for Integrative Medicine in Tucson, sleep disorders are arguably "the most prevalent health concern in the industrialized world."

Sleep is absolutely vital for everything we want to do in life. It's a heightened anabolic state, a time for the growth and rejuvenation of the immune, nervous, skeletal, and muscular systems. Certain restorative genes are turned on only during sleep, brain function and memory consolidation is enhanced, genes promoting myelin formation are turned on, creativity increases, and synapses are strengthened. Not surprisingly, sleep, learning, and mental well-being are tightly linked. Some researchers have even taken to describing sleep as "overnight therapy." If sleep came in a bottle, it would be the most powerful medicine on earth.

But sadly, many of us are tortured by the belief that sleep must come in a single, unbroken block of roughly eight hours. If we fail to reach this benchmark, we conclude that we have a "sleep disorder," a label that mostly serves to increase our anxiety and in turn makes it harder to actually sleep well. But our thinking is flawed. In fact, normal human sleep is probably not monolithic and surely depends on culture and environment. The new thinking is that humans are naturally inclined toward a segmented form of sleep with two distinct phases.

In 2001, historian Roger Ekirch suggested that prior to the modern era, humans slept in two distinct intervals: a "first sleep" from roughly 8 p.m. to midnight and a "second sleep" from 2 a.m. to sunrise, separated by a period of wakefulness that included socializing, quiet time, conversation, and sex. No one expected to sleep through the night.

This pattern probably held for much of human history but began to disappear with the advent of electric lighting. People began to stay up later in the evening as the night became fashionable, and as the Industrial Revolution took hold, sleep gradually morphed into the single block we know today.

Of course, few of us are willing to go to bed at 8 p.m. or adopt a segmented sleeping style, but this history suggests that being awake in the middle of the night may not be a disorder at all. As sleep psychologist Gregg Jacobs put it, "Waking up during the night is part of normal human physiology." The new understanding also tells us that sleep is flexible; there is probably no single right way to sleep.

We're also beginning to suspect that individual variations in sleep patterns probably served an important evolutionary purpose. This is precisely what Elizabeth Marshall Thomas described in her book *The Old Way*. In the wild, the Bushmen (and women) of the Kalahari didn't all go to sleep at the same time or sleep for the same duration. At any given time of the night, someone would be up, tending the fire and minding the camp. Some went to sleep early, others late, and people napped whenever they felt the need. Most importantly, sleep was never stigmatized.

Far from being a problem, this staggered pattern was actually vital to survival. Individual variation meant someone was always up and vigilant, ready to spot predators and spread the alarm. Of course, we no longer worry about being attacked by lions in the middle of the night, but this story of individual variation does put our minds at ease. If your sleeping pattern doesn't happen to fall into line with today's conventional standard, maybe that's simply your personal variation at work; in another time, your sleeping style would have been a valued asset. You probably would have fit right in with a tribe of ancestral hunter–gatherers.

This new–old view of sleep is liberating. We are now free to think of our insomnia, not so much as a disease or an affliction, but as a normal human variation. Above all, it is not something to be ashamed of. The fact that you're awake in the middle of the night may simply be an expression of an ancient physiological inclination. You're awake because the tribe needs you to check the fire and watch for lions. In all likelihood, there's nothing wrong with you or your brain.

SLEEP ACTIVISM AND REFRAMES

By now we've all heard the tips and suggestions for better sleep: no caffeine after noon, make sure your room is dark and cool, and cut back on the screen time before bed. If you're drinking alcohol, do it early and in moderation. These "sleep hygiene" suggestions are sound, but our biggest problem with sleep may well be the way we frame it. If we continue to think of sleep as a selfish act of indulgence that takes us away from our work and family, we'll continue to feel guilty about getting the sleep we truly need.

In *The Sleep Revolution*, Arianna Huffington called for a new sleep ethic and declared that "sleep is a basic human right." This is a step in the right direction, but it's also essential to recognize that sleep is very much a pro-social act. It's a gift to everyone around you and to our world as a whole. When we're rested, we're just easier to get along with. We're more stress tolerant and resilient and we're probably more sensitive to big-picture views of the world. In this sense, sleep is not only pro-health, it's also pro-future. When you head for the couch or off to bed, you're not being lazy and selfish; you're being smart. So do us all a favor and give sleep the respect it deserves.

NATURE AND AWE

Before we can save this world we are losing, we must first learn how to savor what remains.

Terry Tempest Williams

Nature has become a hot topic in the popular health and fitness press and people are commonly advised to get out in nature because "it's good for your health." We're told to practice forest bathing and to be mindfully attentive to the plants, trees and bird life in our urban parks. If we do these practices, our bodies and minds will work better, so the story goes. We'll be more productive, sleep better, focus better and all the rest.

At the same time, we're seeing a surge of interest in the power of awe in human health and psychology. Work by professor Dacher Keltner at UC Berkeley shows that even a mild sense of awe can change attitudes and inspire pro-social behavior. People who watched an awe-inspiring nature video were subsequently more ethical and generous and described themselves as being more connected to others. Keltner's team also found that awe makes people happier and less stressed, even weeks later. Similarly, a study by Jennifer Stellar and Neha John–Henderson found that "positive emotions, especially awe, are associated with lower levels of proinflammatory cytokines."

Research by psychologists at Stanford and the University of Minnesota shows that awe can increase well-being by giving people the sense that they have more time available, a condition known as temporal affluence. Keltner and Jonathan Haidt have even argued that awe is the ultimate collective emotion because it motivates people to do things that enhance the greater good. Research reported in the Journal of Personality and Social Psychology provides empirical support for this claim. The authors found that awe helps people bind to one another, motivating us to act in collaborative ways that enable strong groups and cohesive communities.

All of which sounds like a perfect remedy for our massively stressed-out age. Awe activates the parasympathetic nervous system, which works to calm the fight-or-flight response and dampen the production of toxic stress hormones. It also improves creativity and helps us break out of habitual thinking patterns. In other words, putting ourselves in contact with nature's magnificence is really good for us. We might well say that awe is a form of medicine.

Sadly, modern culture generally fails to appreciate how this works. To be sure, more and more people are going outdoors and trailheads are often packed with cars and people. But not surprisingly, time-in-nature is often presented and even sold to us as something that's good for our personal, individual health. Go out and take a hike because it'll soothe your personal life, heal your body and cure whatever ails you. It'll lower your blood pressure, reduce your blood sugar, maintain your muscle mass and generally make your body work better.

But as usual, this orientation is focused almost entirely on the individual and in that sense, it might even be described as "nature for narcissism." Go out and experience the natural world because it'll make you stronger, fitter, more attractive and all the rest. Harness the power of nature to make a better you. Nature—sometimes described as "Vitamin N"—becomes just another supplement, an aid to personal growth and development. In this view, it inhabits the same category as going to the gym, the juice bar, or the health-food store. Nature exists exclusively for us—to heal us, improve our athletic performance, help us de-stress, be more productive, and all the rest.

Of course, nothing about this orientation comes as much of a surprise, coming as it does from a culture that sees humans as the pinnacle of creation. But from a larger, historical perspective, the whole thing sounds a little too much like an abusive interpersonal relationship. Just imagine an angry, violent partner returning from a bender, seeking solace and comfort from the woman he abused just hours before. Yes, we've brutalized nature for millennia, but now she's going to heal our pain, ease our suffering, and make us whole.

This orientation reaches its apex (or nadir) in the world of adventure sport, where the natural world is simply another thing to be conquered; nature is just another gym, only bigger. Run, climb, bike or swim as fast as you possibly can, dominate the terrain, set some records, and be a champion. In this, nature is nothing more than a platform for our personal greatness. Slowing down and actually experiencing the qualities of the natural world is simply out of the question.

All of which is rather grotesque. If nature is simply a backdrop for our own personal grandeur, it only reinforces our sense of self and in turn separates us further from the world. To really appreciate the totality, the scope and magnificence of the natural world, we've got to be small and we've got to slow down. Nature isn't there *for* us. It's not a tapestry for our personal or species-level greatness. As one quip has it, "You climb the mountain to see the world, not so the world can see you." Or to put it another way, you can't *feel* the awe if you're trying to *be* the awe.

At this point, it helps to step back for a more expansive view. In our historically normal, Paleolithic world, awe was commonplace; the human mind and body were in constant contact with the magnificence and enormity of nature. Thunderstorms and lightning displays were daily events, and animal dramas played out in real time, right before our ancestors' eyes. With no light pollution whatsoever, the night sky would have blazed with an intensity modern humans can scarcely imagine. And around a tribe's local habitat, vast reaches of unknown territory stretched to the horizon, home to whatever our imagination might conjure. On most days, nature filled our ancestors with radical amazement. In other words, awe was a daily feature of life—a universal human experience.

But today, fewer and fewer of us even go outside and when we do, most of our parks are highly domesticated, regulated, noisy, and light polluted. Awe—and the health benefits that come with it—becomes increasingly difficult to come by. We might even say that we're suffering from "awe deprivation." We don't hear much about this condition in the popular press, but judging from the research, it's safe to assume that this is a genuine challenge to public health and a medical condition in its own right. ("Be sure to ask your doctor about awe deprivation.")

THE PRACTICE

As for the art of cultivating awe, there are things that we can do, things that we must do, beginning with going to "the big outside." Get out of yourself and expose yourself to the outrageous, overwhelming power of sky, earth, wind, and water. City parks and green spaces are all well and good, but to really feel the awe, you've got to expose your body and spirit to the enormity of the living earth. Backpacking, river rafting, even extended road trips into remote areas are ideal. Try for one each season, or one every year at least. When it comes to experiencing the awe of the natural world, more is almost always better.

Make yourself vulnerable to the natural world. Go deep into the mountains and spend some nights out. You've going to get some blisters and you're going to get hot, cold, and uncomfortable, but it's all worth it. In the process, try to cultivate a sense of identification with habitat, a continuity between your body and the life around you. Recall the perspective of native and indigenous peoples: "I am the land, the land is me." Can you feel the habitat around you as an extension of your body? Try to see and feel your outdoor world as home, as your original place of belonging.

And, as with any other form of deep engagement, it's essential that we leave distractions behind, especially the greatest distraction of all, the smart phone. The mere presence of the device, even in the unlikely event that it's turned off, distorts the experience. In fact, taking your phone out on a hike is best described as *phubbing* the natural world (from phone + snubbing), as in "my immediate convenience is more important than the awesome reality of creation."

So yes, of course, go outside and spend time in nature, but don't expect it to transform you automatically or passively, without effort. The pleasant sensations are all well and good, but it's essential that we go deeper. Imagine the continuities that exist between your body and the life around you. Sit quietly and feel your kinship with life. Forget the modern world and let your mind drift back in time, millions of years to the era of ancestral unity, the Great Integrity of the Taoist tradition. Shrink your profile and imagine yourself as an intimate participant in the natural processes around you. Ultimately, this is where the power lies. As the deep ecologist Arne Næss put it, "The smaller we come to feel ourselves compared to the mountain, the nearer we come to participating in its greatness."

DEGROWTH

> We are in the beginning of a mass extinction, and all you can talk about is money and fairy tales of eternal economic growth.
>
> Greta Thunberg

> If you know when you have enough, you are wealthy.
>
> Lao Tzu
> *Tao te Ching*

Our next practice has to do with the material world, our possessions and in particular, our relationship to the idea of growth. Sometimes described as minimalism or essentialism, this practice is a sensible, practical response to the dominant, future-hostile ideology of modern times.

As many of us have come to recognize in recent years, the belief in unlimited economic growth lies at the heart of our predicament. Political pundits, commentators, and economists typically tell us that growth is a cure-all for whatever ails us, growth is always for the good of everyone, a rising tide lifts all boats, and on it goes. In short, growthism is baked into our economic system and the psychology of the modern world.

But uncontrolled growth violates everything we know about animal physiology and ecosystem function. When economies grow relentlessly, nature is always the loser. Growing the economy while simultaneously undermining the ecological base that supports it is doomed to fail. Some have called it a Ponzi scheme, a suicidal economy, an extinction economy. And as Edward Abbey famously put it, "Growth is the ideology of the cancer cell."

All of which is fueled by one of the most perverse metrics in the modern human experience: Gross Domestic Product. As many observers have pointed out, GDP measures *all* economic activity, even activity that's contrary to human and biospheric health. As a metric, it isn't even close to being humane or ecologically sound. All it measures is raw activity, no matter the quality.

Thankfully, an increasingly vocal minority is pushing back against growthism with a new discipline called degrowth economics or simply degrowth. The core idea is to scale back all non-essential economic activity, to contract the human footprint to something more proportional and appropriate. Advocates include Jason Hickel, author of *Less is More: How Degrowth Will Save the World*. Some call on us to "depave, debuild, deconstruct" while others call for a "graceful collapse" that includes less fossil-fueled activity, less meat consumption, less conventional affluence, and more of what really matters: time in contact with our life-supporting systems of people and habitat.

To make this happen, advocates call for a reversal of the wealth pump that robs from the less fortunate. In essence, the goal is to tax and shame the affluent and use their resources to support the basic, fundamental, human-scale flourishing of the less fortunate. In one sense at least, degrowth economics couldn't be simpler. It requires no fancy economic theories, research, think tanks or exploratory committees. Just go back to the original Robin Hood.

THE PRACTICE OF MINIMALISM

Degrowth sounds intriguing, but it also sounds like an extremely heavy lift for society and modern culture. After all, most of us have been systematically trained, almost from birth, to believe in the promise of more. To degrow our current economy to the extent required would require a massive shift in human and cultural psychology, not to mention a tectonic shift in modern political discourse.

Of course, some people now say that degrowth is inevitable no matter what; one way or another human impact is going to be drastically reduced—we can do it voluntarily, or we can do it catastrophically. But in any case, there's nothing to stop us from practicing degrowth as individuals. As activists, we may not be able to stop the mad, compulsive, cultural pursuit of growth, but we can degrow our own lives and in the process, make ourselves happier and more relevant.

All of which will require a substantial shift in our assumptions and mind-set. Trained by consumer culture and the prevailing ideology of growthism, we're quick to assume that personal degrowth is going to mean adversity, pain, and suffering. If more is more, then less must be less. If affluence is good, minimalism must be bad. To the average ear, minimalism sounds like austerity, even poverty. Thanks, but no thanks.

But this is simply a failure of our imagination. In fact, minimalism is actually a pathway to more of what really matters; more freedom from possession, more control, more free time, and more opportunity for creative work. When we stop buying so much stuff, we suddenly have a lot more room in our lives for the important things. In other words, minimalism is not austerity and it's not poverty—it's simply a better way to live. Think of it as an affluence of less. To put it another way, minimalism is actually a path to a new world of abundance. Without a mountain of possessions to be managed, your sense of wealth can actually grow.

JUDGMENT CALLS

Of course, none of this is easy. Minimalism is a powerful path, but modern life often forces us into nearly impossible dilemmas and judgment calls on consumption and impact. Like it or not, we're embedded in a fossil-fueled world, a tyrannical system that's been massively developed for human convenience and corporate profit. And if we want to do anything at all in this world, we have no choice but to participate to some degree. Almost everything we do now requires computers, electricity, transportation, plastics, and even some level of industrial agriculture. You can try to live and function at an Amish level of impact, but it's going to be a struggle.

Naturally, all of this causes us even more stress as it gums up our thinking. You want to go for a hike because it's good for your mind and body, but you've got to burn a tank of gas to get there. Your house needs repairs, but there are no sustainable solutions. You want to wear a T-shirt promoting your cause, but it's made from non-organic cotton, printed on the other side of the world. You've got to wear shoes, but it's almost impossible to find a pair that isn't made with toxic materials and dubious labor practices.

Every day a thousand judgment calls and micro-decisions. We study the options but the homework is overwhelming and often inconclusive, and if we choose the easier, higher-impact path, we wind up feeling guilty. All of which leads to folly and even paralysis. How much homework can we put into these choices without going completely crazy? How much should we participate in the toxic system in order to fight the toxic system?

The reality is excruciating: Sometimes we have to use fossil fuels to put a stop to fossil fuels. Sometimes we have to use the products of industrial civilization to put the brakes on industrial civilization. And even worse perhaps, sometimes we have to use the advertising, media and publicity practices of a toxic culture to shine a light on its toxicity. As author Nathan John Hagens has put it, sometimes we have to "use the devil's tools to do Gaia's work".

We grapple with the dilemmas as best we can, but perhaps there's a better way to navigate these choices, beginning with a series of questions. Think of the consumption or impact dilemma you're facing, then ask yourself:

Does my action contribute in any plausible way to the future health of the natural world?

Does it serve my life-supporting systems?

Is it beneficial for my body?

Does it plausibly support the long-term viability of habitat or the welfare of my tribe and community?

Does it help create a sense of meaning and purpose for me and the people around me?

If the answer is no, move on. If the answer is yes, do it and feel good about it. The decision has been made and there's no sense feeling remorse or guilt.

Along the way, it also helps to reconsider our values and identity. Most importantly, it's essential that we stop glorifying conventional, material affluence. In short, stop worshiping the rich. Stop with the belief that rich people are somehow smarter, better, and harder working than everyone else. All of this is utter nonsense. Beyond the point of optima, excess luxury is an embarrassment, possibly even a crime—definitely not something to aspire to.

Likewise, stop identifying with your possessions. In other words, *you are not your stuff.* The continued growth of the consumeristic machine depends, not just on fossil fuels and plastics, but on large numbers of people identifying with the things that they own. But owning a shiny object does not make you a shiny person. If you want to identify with something, identify with the natural world, your life-support systems, your social circles, or your work.

We may not be able to avoid using and benefiting from carbon-intensive transport, industrial agriculture, or other forms of Earth-hostile behavior, but we can always do it with attention and awareness. Do these things as you must, but understand that when you do, you're participating in a highly destructive, future-hostile activity. Keep your attention open and don't be lulled back into the consumeristic trance.

Likewise, don't let the perfect become the enemy of the good. In theory, you might be able to get your fossil-fueled impact and plastic consumption down to almost zero, but if you hamstring your mobility and your activism in the process, it might all be for nothing. Better to go towards balance and proportion, which is to say, art.

KEEP A BEAT

The final practice has to do with rhythmic engagement with the world, an oscillation of effort and attention, even in the face of overwhelming demands on our time and energy. As you'll see, this practice is absolutely vital to function, effectiveness, and even survival itself.

Looking at the frenetic pace of commercial and industrial activity in the modern world, what we see is something that looks very much like a chronic disease, a relentless assault on our life-supporting systems and, in turn, our bodies and our spirits. In every minute of every day, massive amounts of carbon are being pumped into the atmosphere, species are being forced out of their homes, oceans are being over-fished, forests are being cut down, soil and groundwater are being depleted, mountaintops are being "removed," and minerals are being strip-mined. The destruction never sleeps.

All of which is not just depressing, it also poses a massive challenge for the health and sanity of the activist: When we realize the chronic nature of the destruction, we're tempted to answer with our own chronic efforts. If the destruction never stops, neither should we, so we double down and triple down on our efforts. More meetings, more homework, more actions, more time at the keyboard. We triage out the nonessentials and devote ever more energy to the fight.

It's honorable work, but it's also contrary to our ancestral experience and the deep nature of our bodies. For tens of thousands of years, our ancestors thrived on an oscillating pattern of engagement and rest. Go for a hunt or a walkabout and expose yourself to the elements for a few days, then return to camp to relax. Push your body hard, then give yourself time to heal up.

In their 1988 book *The Paleolithic Prescription*, anthropologists S. Boyd Eaton, Marjorie Shostak, and Melvin Konner described this pattern of engagement and resting as "the Paleolithic rhythm." Without question, this pattern is the norm for human beings. Even well into the age of agriculture, natural light ruled human activity and people lived a rhythmic lifestyle. There can be no question that this kind of oscillation kept us strong and resilient.

The pattern is easy to understand. Hunting, exploration, and adventure is a time of fight-flight activation. The autonomic nervous system goes into high gear, providing the physical resources we need to run, walk long distances, climb trees and ford rivers. All of which can cause plenty of physical injury, both subtle and acute, but back in camp, everything in the body goes the other way as the rest-digest cycle kicks in. Surrounded by family, friends, food and gossip, the body eases back into a healing, parasympathetic state. No hurry, you've got long days to rest up and rejuvenate.

For the activist, this model offers a challenge and a paradoxical lesson. Yes, our predicament is a genuine emergency that demands radical action and sustained, even desperate effort. And yes, it's hard to relax when you know the devastation that's going on just outside your door. But it's also true that we've got to keep our strength up. You won't be of much use to anyone if you burn up your body and spirit with chronic effort. On the contrary, you'll flame out and lapse back into the quagmire of exhaustion, depression, and despair. Every athletic coach knows how this works: intensive training must always oscillate with deep rest. Otherwise, the effort is wasted.

All of which argues for a high-contrast lifestyle of engagement and down time. Look for an athletic lifestyle: fight the fight as best you can, then allow your body to heal up. Engage your adversary, then retreat to a safe haven. Focus as intensely as possible, then give your time and attention over to deep relaxation. Forget the conventional pace of modern culture and the always-on demands of digital life. Rest is not some kind of failure, nor is it a sign of sloth or weakness. Rather, it's fundamental to function and an essential gift that we give to the world.

SAPIENCE

Find your place on the planet. Dig in, and take
responsibility from there.

Gary Snyder
The Practice of the Wild

As we've seen, our encounter with The Knowledge ex-
poses us to a series of rude awakenings and shocks to
our equanimity. Climate, biosphere, habitat destruction,
social and economic injustice; the list is familiar by now.
But there's yet another bitter pill that we must swallow, the
realization that modern culture shows a striking absence
of reflection and introspection about the big questions of
life and the human experience.

Looking across human history over the last several thousand years, we see a wide range of wisdom cultures that
have actively sought integration, harmony, and health.
Native and indigenous cultures, Buddhism, mystical traditions and major religions have all sought sapience (as in
Homo sapiens) in one form or another. These cultures have
actively supported individual efforts at wise living, proportion, beauty, and what Michael Dowd called "a right
relationship to reality." And far from being exceptional or

unusual, this orientation towards wisdom, contemplation, and right living has been commonplace and even unremarkable in our history; a genuine human universal.

By comparison, we now live in what might well be described as a "non-wisdom culture" or even an "anti-wisdom culture." In many ways, our priorities and values are antithetical to integration and even survival itself. This disconnect is revealed in what modern society holds to be sacred: money, wealth, material affluence, productivity and performance, efficiency, speed, convenience, power and control, status, celebrity and fame. These are the things that we value above all else.

To put it another way, we're worshiping the wrong things. A quick Internet search tells the story: almost a million hits for "the economy is sacred" but a mere handful of results for "the biosphere is sacred." Disgraced former president Donald Trump even referred to the Dow Jones Industrial Average as "a sacred number." So it's no wonder that we're floundering. It's no wonder that we're paralyzed when attempting to move the needle on our eco-social crisis; our culture is working against us and we're philosophically unequipped to do what needs to be done.

In fact, most of us would be hard-pressed to identify or describe what a wisdom orientation actually consists of. We're practical minded, focused on tangible, financial rewards at the end of our efforts. We believe in the power of intelligence, but we never took a course in wisdom and have little to say about the matter. And when it comes to *sapience*, most of us will come up empty handed; we might even wonder if it's even relevant to anything.

But far from being some kind of fuzzy, abstract, intellectual concept promoted by long-dead philosophers, wisdom is not only relevant, but extremely practical, especially in the face of overwhelming existential threats.

So the question looms: If wisdom is such a desirable quality of human experience, why do we fail to teach it? Why is it that modern students can go through an entire educational journey and never be exposed to these foundational ideas? Why don't we start at the beginning and teach children the fundamentals of sapience? Why do we wait until college-level philosophy courses? Shouldn't wisdom be integrated into education at every level? If we're ever going to exercise sapience as a people, we're going to have to start teaching it, or at least making the effort.

INTERDEPENDENCE

There is urgency in coming to see the world as a web of interrelated processes of which are integral parts, so that all of our choices and actions have consequences for the world around us.

Alfred North Whitehead

Without question, one of the most enduring themes in wisdom cultures is the recognition and appreciation of interdependence in living things. No matter the tradition, life is viewed as a unified tensegrity structure—a bicycle wheel if you will—in which every part is dependent on every other part. Nothing stands alone.

A selection from cultures around the world shows a near-universal interest in themes of interdependence and continuity:

The Zen tradition: "To your way of thinking, your skin is a thing which separates and protects you from the outside world. To my way of thinking, my skin is a thing which connects me and opens me to the outside world, which in any case is not the outside world."

Zen philosopher Alan Watts: "You and I are all as much continuous with the physical universe as a wave is continuous with the ocean." Likewise, "...civilized human beings are alarmingly ignorant of the fact that they are continuous with their natural surroundings. It is as necessary to have air, water, plants, insects, birds, fish and mammals as it is to have brains, hearts, lungs and stomachs. The former are our external organs in the same way the latter are our internal organs."

Thich Nhat Hanh: "True self is non-self, the awareness that the self is made only of non-self elements. There's no separation between self and other, and everything is interconnected. Once you are aware of that you are no longer caught in the idea that you are a separate entity."

Zen master Yasutani Roshi (1885-1973): "The fundamental delusion of humanity is to suppose that I am here and you are out there."

Carl Jung: "My self is not confined to my body. It extends into all the things I have made and all the things around me...Everything surrounding me is part of me."

John Muir: "When we try to pick out anything by itself, we find it hitched to everything else in the universe. One fancies a heart like our own must be beating in every crystal and cell..."

Likewise, the Lakota people of North America say *mi-takuye oyasin*, a phrase that translates as "all my relations." It's a prayer of oneness with all forms of life: people, animals, birds, insects, trees, and plants, and even rocks, rivers, mountains, and valleys.

We've heard these non-dual, all-is-one declarations many times, but we're often quick to dismiss them as the musings of inspired, romantic, but unrealistic minds. So we return to our daily lives mostly unaffected, our familiar perceptions and dualities intact. One-world consciousness is for poets and dreamers, not for normal people with busy lives.

But it turns out that these writers, mystics, and scientists are not just musing about some utopian, aspirational, make-believe world. Rather, their observations reveal a biological, psychological, and spiritual truth. Today, a mountain of scientific research confirms the continuities between our bodies, our minds, our fellows, and our habitat. These are not separate, self-contained things; they are truly continuous with one another. Feel it or not, we are literally kin with the world.

In fact, continuity is what sustains us. As leaves on a vast tree, we are utterly dependent on the branches, trunk, and roots. When we fail to appreciate our connection with the rest of creation, we leave ourselves isolated, vulnerable, anxious, and afraid. It's no wonder that so many wisdom traditions advocate for some idea of karma and consequence. In a radically interconnected biological and social world, how could it be otherwise? Don't expect to abuse the biosphere and habitat without effect. Don't expect to abuse human and non-human animals without consequences. It is continuity that sustains us, just as much as food, water, and air. Continuity is the essence of life.

THE WISDOM OF THE INVERSE U

> For all objects and experiences, there is a quantity that has optimum value. Above that quantity, the variable becomes toxic. To fall below that value is to be deprived.
>
> Ecologist Gregory Bateson

Another universal theme in wisdom traditions revolves around what today we call the inverse U curve. If you've ever taken a course in biology, physiology, health sciences, or even engineering, you've seen it a thousand times. In every natural system, from cellular metabolism to the large-scale interactions in ecosystems, there's always a Goldilocks zone, a sweet spot between *hyper* and *hypo*, a rising curve of benefit, followed by a tipping point, diminishing returns, and a downward arc that leads to systemic failure, ill health, or worse.

So it's no surprise to see a similar idea throughout wisdom traditions around the world. The ancient Greeks—Aristotle, Plato, and Socrates in particular—talked about the "golden mean." As they saw it, "Measure and proportion manifest themselves in all areas of beauty and virtue." Meanwhile, on the other side of the planet, Chinese philosophers Lao Tzu, Chuang Tzu, and Confucius spoke about "the doctrine of the mean." The Buddha himself likened right living to having just the right amount of tension on the strings of a musical instrument. Even the three bears understood that the one in the middle is "just right."

Examples are everywhere in the natural sciences. We see sweet spots for food consumption, protein, minerals, alcohol, salt, antioxidants, and even water. And it's not just biochemistry. Researchers have even found a sweet spot for the "protective effects of adversity" in childhood; too hard is detrimental to the child's development, but so is too easy. And as we've seen, there are optimal levels of stress for the human animal; a little is good for body and spirit, but go past the sweet spot and we begin to suffer.

Every physician knows that there's a *hypo* and a *hyper* for every treatment. Every physical therapist knows that there's a sweet spot for range of motion in skeletal joints. Every endocrinologist knows that there's an ideal level for hormones in the human body. Every athletic trainer knows that there's a sweet spot between over and under training. Every music teacher, every massage therapist, every craftsperson, every artist; if there was ever a universal principle for crafting a successful human life, this is it.

But sadly, modern culture simply hasn't gotten the message on this score, or to be more precise, we simply ignore it. Driven by relentless marketing and ever more sophisticated advertising, everything is now exaggerated and hyperbolic. More is always more and there are no limits to anything; no optimal levels, no sweet spots, no tipping points and no domain of diminishing returns. It's all one rising curve of benefit and profit that goes on forever.

In other words, we've managed to convince ourselves that we're exempt from the general principles that govern everything else in the living world, all of which drives us into a frenzy of activity that further distances us from the natural processes that keep us alive. Any ecologist can see this as foolish, arrogant, and even suicidal. For anyone with any sense of proportion, this must be obvious.

For example, consider what the inverse U curve means for possession. It's easy to see how the curve implies a sense of proportion and what we might call "enoughness." In fact, such an affluence-benefit curve should behave just like every other inverse U curve in the human experience. On the left side of the curve we meet the simple animal needs of food, shelter, decent clothing, a noble livelihood and competent medical care. On this side, there are huge payoffs in personal satisfaction and happiness.

But beyond the sweet spot, affluence fails to deliver. Private jets, second homes, high fashion, and a thousand gadgets: these things look great in the advertisements, but don't measure up to the hype. We're conditioned to think of these things as attractive, even beautiful, but in the context of planetary destruction they must be seen for what they are: ugly, wasteful, and embarrassing.

Ultimately, the inverse U is so prevalent across the natural world that it makes sense to use it as a general principle for living. The curve gives us guidance and powerful, practical life lessons that we can use in virtually everything we do, including our activism and our martial artistry. When in doubt, seek the sweet spot.

NATURAL ACTIVISM

> Wise people succeed because they never force an outcome.
>
> Lao Tzu
> *Tao te Ching*

Interdependence, integration, inverse U curves—what do these ideas have to say about our practice of activism? Is there a way to make our engagement consistent with the qualities of the living world itself? Is there a form of activism that mimics natural systems, physiology and ecosystem dynamics?

In fact, such an orientation exists and the good news is that we don't have to re-invent the wheel. Long ago, the Taoists of ancient China described a practice of skill in action as *wu-wei*, or "effortless action." In this tradition, skill was a great organizing theme for living. Nothing is forced; when the artist works in harmony with her body and surroundings, movement and action come forth without friction or effort. Living in the sweet spot of engagement, she seeks the optima in all things, all actions, all relations. As an agent working in cooperation with nature, she looks for opportune moments and acts with a sense of balance and proportion. This is the ultimate expression of mastery.

Just as with skill in any other domain, natural activism would be effortless. We imagine the seasoned, skillful artivist navigating complex terrain, power dynamics, impossible dilemmas and doing it all with little apparent effort. No matter the ambiguity, chaos, or complexity of her situation, she adjusts and adapts on the fly, finding sweet spots in engagement, pace, intensity, activity, and above all, relationship.

It may sound like a fantasy or magic, but it's not. The practice relies on focused, concentrated attention to surroundings and circumstance. To act effortlessly in the world, you've got to feel the world, especially the patterns, rhythms, and pace of activity. For the ancient Taoists, this meant listening to the subtle features of nature, but today the situation is more demanding. Not only must we attend to natural processes that are increasingly under assault, we must also pay attention to the myriad actions and relationships in the social and political world. It's a tall order, but necessary nonetheless.

All of which tells us something vital about stress. For the natural activist, stress is not a beast to be conquered or eliminated, but a vital form of information; it tells her when she's deviating from the path of effortless action and skill. The beginner ignores her stress until it screams out for attention, but the master feels its earliest, most subtle beginnings. With experience and training, she learns to feel the frictions earlier and earlier, as whispers of sensation that creep into the process. Never something to be ignored or resisted, it's an essential guide to natural engagement.

But make no mistake. *Wu-wei* is not about passivity, weakness or submission. It's not about avoiding conflict or retreating to the familiar. It's about skillful action no matter the circumstances. Some situations call for intensity and commitment, but even in the act of passionate engagement, the artist still seeks the flow natural movement, balance and proportion.

This is the Taoist ideal: *Wu-wei* in all actions, across our lives. To put it another way, skill isn't just for athletics or music or the professions; it's for the everyday things, the chores, the routine tasks that we tend to ignore. The challenge is to practice skill in all things. Focus your concentrated effort at the beginning of the learning process, then relinquish that effort gradually until nothing but effortless action remains.

SACRED RAGE, INDIGENOUS PATIENCE

Don't trust anyone who isn't angry.

John Trudell
Native American author, poet, and activist

When we think of a wise person, most of us imagine someone who's calm, tranquil, and relaxed, even in the face of outrageous challenges. Rarely do we think of someone who's angry, and in fact we're quick to assume that anger is the mark of impulsivity and poor character.

And yet, this assumption is misleading. Why would the wise ones reject a basic human emotion? Wise people are human beings after all, and isn't anger a fundamental part of the human animal's emotional repertoire? All mammals share this trait in some degree, and we can be sure that it gave us some kind of survival advantage throughout our history. In fact, transcending anger would seem to be a fool's goal, akin to transcending our ability to feel love, passion, curiosity, or wonder.

Unfortunately, many of us in the modern world feel uncomfortable with anger and do whatever we can to make it go away. Prevailing cultural belief holds that anger is a character flaw, even a personality disorder. If you're angry, there's something wrong with you that needs to be managed, extinguished or dampened by practice and self-control. If you're angry, you need an anger-management course, therapy and/or medication. In particular, you need a more powerful pre-frontal cortex to bring all that nastiness under strict neurological control. If your hair is on fire, you need to put the fire out.

But what if we're wrong about all of this? What if anger is a normal human-animal response to wickedly abnormal circumstances and an alien environment? What if your anger is an appropriate, rational, life-affirming response to the destruction of life-supporting habitat? And what if the *absence* of anger is the real the dysfunction of our age?

So perhaps a distinction is in order. On one hand, our ordinary, garden-variety anger is simply a stress-driven response to cognitive overload, temporal poverty, or ego boundary violations. It's impulsive, mostly unconscious, and not particularly functional. It's often dangerous, both to the rager herself and those around her. And even worse, it's disintegrating to mind, spirit, and body. So yes, this kind of anger is something to be avoided.

But then there's the "sacred rage" described by Native American author John Trudell and others. This is the fire that burns in the face of persistent injustice and oppression. It's a mature, sophisticated form of anger: purpose and value driven, sincere, patient, dignified, and maybe even inspirational. Observing, witnessing, lying in wait for the right opportunity, it pulls the body together and powers it through outrageous challenges. There's no overt expression, no loss of control, no outbursts, only focused, intentional and persistent action.

This kind of anger is a reflection of our values, our attention and a healthy concern for what we hold dear. As Edward Abbey put it, "Love implies anger. The man who is angered by nothing cares about nothing." And if you love habitat—as indigenous, historically-normal humans do—then you ought to be furious when it's threatened or destroyed outright. In this sense, anger is perfectly healthy and appropriate.

This kind of rage is a sacred expression of our animal nature and our fight for life. Even our anxiety, depression, doubts and confusion are vital. As the writer and eco-therapist Joanna Macy put it, "The sorrow, grief, and rage you feel is a measure of your humanity and your evolutionary maturity." Likewise, author Chris Hedges: "If you do not feel profound grief over the coming ecocide, you are shutting your eyes to reality. Grief is an emotional, physical and spiritual necessity—the price you pay for love."

But rage, we might say, is not enough. It becomes even more powerful when coupled with a complimentary sense of patience and reserve. And on reflection, we realize that this must be the historical norm for most of the human species. After all, for the vast, overwhelming majority of our time on this Earth, our only sense of urgency was in response to episodic natural events. Go fast when there's a wildfire, bad weather, or an encounter with wild animals, but otherwise, there's simply no hurry. Why would there be? Just take your time.

Not surprisingly, indigenous people seem to have a much deeper appreciation for the long view, both past and future. Native culture reinforces an appreciation for ancestry, history, and what we might call deep time. In this long view, there's less need to panic, even in the face of epic, looming catastrophe. Yes, there's vital work to be done, but time will take care of everything. Yes, the anger still burns, be we can also be calm. Call it "indigenous patience" if you will; this is the normal human condition.

This insight gives us some relief and maybe even a sense of peace. Maybe it's not really necessary to spend our modern days in a state of chronic urgency and angst. Maybe we can relax back into our normal human state of being. So take a breath. Our ecosocial crisis is what it is. There's nothing to be gained by running amok in a state of manic, frenetic activity. Take the long view.

UNITE TO SURVIVE

> Action, as distinguished from fabrication, is never possible in isolation; to be isolated is to be deprived of the capacity to act.
>
> Hannah Arendt
> *The Human Condition*

As we've seen, the human animal does not and cannot live in isolation. We are hyper-social primates after all, constantly sharing our experiences, our emotions, our sense of meaning and our values. And since our health is co-created, it stands to reason that our sapience—or lack of thereof—would be co-created as well.

For the activist and the artivist, this implies a strategy and a way to live. Radically over-matched by powerful adversaries, our only chance for effectiveness lies in our ability to work together, to seek out others, build community and relationships. In short, collaboration is good for the movement and good for our health; we are stronger together. Our various tribes and communities are like tensegrity structures in which each element contributes to the strength of the whole.

Seeking out others is also a powerful stress strategy. There's solid neurobiology here and some have suggested that this "tend and befriend response" is another option for people under stress. Yes, we can fight or flee, but we're also inclined to seek out one another, share our experiences, and in the process, find some measure of relief. There's no question that this social contact and sense of belonging is a genuine form of medicine in its own right.

The emerging disciplines of social neuroscience and interpersonal neurobiology show how tightly our bodies are bound to our social experience. In effect, we are constantly co-regulating one another's autonomic nervous systems via what's been described as a "resonance circuit." Mirror neurons in the brain light up in response to other people's posture and facial expressions. In turn, this information is relayed down the vagus nerve to the gut for more processing where in essence, it allows us to run emotional simulations of what other people around us are feeling. From there, information is relayed back up to the brain where it contributes to the remodeling of the prefrontal cortex, shaping our attention and ultimately our behavior.

Incredible as this system is, it's also not really surprising, given our naked vulnerability in prehistory. As we've seen, humans on the grassland we're constantly exposed to predation and with no claws to protect us, the best strategy was gang up and stay together. Naturally, this kind of survival pressure favored tribes that were intensely social. Those who could read one another's emotions, postures, and facial expressions would have been at a distinct advantage. Likewise, tribes that emphasized social equity and a level hierarchy would have fared much better when exposed to the challenges of survival.

It's no surprise therefore that a powerful pro-social identification shows up in many indigenous and Eastern cultures. This is most conspicuous in the African philosophy of *ubuntu*. (pronounced uu-boon-too) According to this perspective, there exists a common bond between all human beings and it is through this bond that we discover our own human qualities; we affirm our humanity when we acknowledge the humanity of others.

For native people, identity is never independent—it's interdependent, intimately connected to the life and welfare of the tribe, the family, the community. People define themselves not as individuals but as participants in a larger social order. As the bushmen of South Africa put it, "We are people through other people" and "I am what I am because of who we are."

All of which suggests that the ideal strategy is to avoid division and build relationships whenever possible. Fighting and conflict will always be part of the human experience, but the antidote is to focus on the biology, the psychology, and lived experience of the human animal—the human universals. Ultimately, everyone on the planet is animated by the same basic needs and desires. Everyone, regardless of party affiliation, ideology, or culture, wants comfort, food and water, to be surrounded by good people and to have some meaningful work. No one wants a dysfunctional future, no one wants their children to suffer extreme weather, droughts, food insecurity, or war.

To be sure, it's important to talk about perpetrators and the various advantages and disadvantages of different philosophies for action, but at the end of the day, it's essential to remember the power of the human universals. Speak to the totality of humanity. As Extinction Rebellion puts it, "Unite to Survive." So stay in touch, find your people and keep them close.

CREATE FORWARD, HEAL FORWARD

> Life can only be understood backwards, but it
> must be lived forwards.
>
> Søren Kierkegaard

If we're going to exercise sapience in the face of extreme circumstance, we've got to be pointed in the right direction—which is to say, forward—but unfortunately, we often get this wrong at the outset. When something goes wrong in our lives, our common impulse is to find a solution by going back to the original condition, whatever that happened to be.

In other words, when the going gets tough, most of us revert to the familiar. Traumas big and small come into our lives, and we long to regain the sense of control, predictability, and wholeness that we experienced in days gone by. We tell our friends that we're going to "get back in shape" and we dream about returning to our former state of youthful vigor and exuberance. Likewise, we imagine degraded ecosystems bouncing back to their original, old-growth glory after being raped by strip-mining, clear-cutting, and development. It's no wonder we see a growing industry of resilience training in education, business, community settings, and leadership. Everyone wants to go back.

But our thinking is flawed. The river of physiology and ecosystem function only flows forward, and it's never the same river twice. Strictly speaking, there can be no bouncing back for any living systems, bodies or habitats. Healing does occur, but when it does, it's always a transformation to some new state of integration. The thing we call resilience is really a creative process of moving forward.

Suppose you suffer a sporting injury. With rest and treatment you usually get over it, and you might even suppose that you're "back to normal." But the tissue in question is different than before; your body has engineered a workaround and some compensations—some scar tissue, some thickening of fibers, maybe some new neural stimulation to your muscular system. Your body works well enough now and it no longer gives you pain, but in essence, it's really a different body. You haven't bounced back—you've bounced forward.

The same holds true for habitat. When a forest ecosystem burns or is clear-cut, it eventually transforms to a new state of function and maybe even health. We might say it "heals," but conditions are never precisely the same; some species have disappeared and new ones have taken hold. Given enough time, the forest grows again and may even appear to have recovered, but there are subtle new relationships between plants, animals, and microorganisms.

The problem with our popular image of resilience is that it offers a false hope of return. We lead ourselves to believe we can rebound to a golden age when everything was working "as nature intended." All our modern "re" words suffer a similar flaw: return, restore, rebound, rebuild, rewild, regenerate, recuperate. The belief is seductive: with good luck and hard work, we can take the broken pieces, repair them, put them back into their original order, and everything will be "as good as new." But belief in this kind of resilience can blind us to the creative actions we need to move forward. Even worse, it can leave us feeling hopeless. If going back is impossible, then there's nothing left but to suffer.

This forward-leaning orientation might sound like a strategy for occasional use, especially in the wake of trauma, injury, or disease, but when we take the lesson to heart, we start looking at our lives and our activism from a whole new perspective. In this, creating and healing forward becomes a fundamental skill in its own right, something we can practice every day, always working with what we've got on hand, continuously putting together new combinations that move us ahead. In this practice, healing and creating forward becomes a muscle that gets stronger with use. The more we create with existing conditions, the better we get.

IT'S ALL MUSCLE

In fact, repetition is always the name of the game, no matter the challenge. In the popular imagination, activism is usually thought of as a kind of special case, an oddball activity in the world of human affairs—nothing more than a bunch of angry discontents with an axe to grind. But in fact, activism can be thought of as a skill like any other, not altogether different from athletics, music, dance, or craft. It's the product of a plastic human nervous system, learning and growing with repetition and experience.

To be completely accurate, we might go so far as to describe activism as a meta-skill, a collection of subskills that add up to proficiency in the larger effort. The serious activist or artivist will want to master language arts, as well as the intricacies of government, policy, social psychology, leadership, and personal development; there's a lot of material to learn. Nevertheless, the point remains; all of these elements will follow the same familiar principle of every human art and skill—that is, practice is everything.

All of which is solid ground in the world of athletic training where every experienced coach knows the master principle: development of the mind-body is *always* specific to the challenge imposed on the athlete. Stress the body with weight training, running, climbing, or cycling, and it will respond with incredibly precise adaptations to support further instances of that activity. The transformation is always specific, which is to say, there are no fancy tricks involved. If you want to get better at a task, practice doing *exactly* that task.

Every neuroscientist in the world understands how this works. That is, microscopic changes to the brain are almost always use-dependent. Synapses, myelin sheaths, and even the sensory-motor cortex of the brain itself; all follow the same principle, strengthening circuitry in anticipation of upcoming encounters with the challenge in question. In other words, experience is the master sculptor of our bodies and in turn, our lives and behavior.

Strictly speaking, activism isn't precisely the same as athletic training. It's a little less muscular and a little more psycho-spiritual. It's less about producing powerful physical movement and more about social persuasion, education, and influence. Nevertheless, it makes sense to suppose that active engagement would follow the same use-it-to-develop-it principles as athletics, music, or any other skill. How could it be otherwise?

Put yourself into contact with society and culture, and you'll get better at precisely that. Take a risk by going outside your comfort zone and you'll get better at precisely that. Expose yourself to the uncertainty and ambiguity of public speaking, writing, protest, and civil disobedience and you'll improve your performance in these domains. To put it another way, engagement is a learnable skill and the way to get good at it is by doing more of it.

At first, your engagement with the world will be tentative and even scary. The social exposure is intimidating and you may be tempted to shrink back from the challenge. But this is the time to think like a coach, an athlete, a musician, or a neuroscientist. The path to success built on repetition. What kind of specific adaptations would you like to create? Every action, every public presentation, every difficult meeting or phone call, every organizational meeting—these are your reps. Put in the time and your body will respond.

Of course you'll be awkward in the beginning. You're going to stumble, say the wrong thing, mis-read adversaries and allies, mis-interpret circumstances, and spread confusion in the process. It's not going to feel good and you're going to feel like giving up. But have faith in the process. Rest assured that your body understands, even if you don't. It's an invisible but extremely powerful process that's millions of years old. Your body will feel the repetition in your experience and start building new tissue and circuitry to make the next series easier. You might well feel like you're floundering, but you can trust your nervous system to do the work. Keep showing up and your skill will grow.

COACHES, LEADERS AND ELDERS

As we've seen, the modern activist is faced us with an overwhelming set of wicked problems, complexity, cognitive overload, moral dilemmas, and just plain confusion.

Even on the best days, it's not an easy path and we're likely to wonder what to make of it all. Surely there must be someone out there who can lead us out of the swamp and into something resembling a functional future.

But sadly, almost no one in power is stepping up in any truly significant or relevant way. Conventional politics is gummed up with petty bickering, useless turf battles and posturing, and many players are simply lining their pockets while perpetuating the status quo. With few exceptions, there's no real effort to go upstream to the root of our various dysfunctions. And even worse, there's a almost willful refusal to talk about what really matters. Almost no one in power is talking about biology, life-supporting systems, the natural world or even human universals.

This is why activists and artivists must be prepared to step into the leadership vacuum. Like it or not, ready for it or not, it's up to us to point the way towards some kind of functional future, some kind of path towards truth, compassion, and health. In this sense, activists must come to see themselves, not just as political agents, but as teachers, leaders, coaches, and even tribal elders.

All of which calls for another look back in history. As we've seen, humans have spent most of their time on Earth in wild, outdoor, predator-rich habitats. Conditions were sometimes dangerous and aside from having a rich oral tradition, there was no guidebook for making a living. When times were hard, people naturally looked to the elders for guidance. Should we go upriver or down? Should we move our camp? Should we hunt in the distant valley or stay close to our familiar territory? Surely the wise ones would know what to do.

This is why respect for elders is universal in native and

indigenous cultures. This is also why servant leadership is often held to be the ultimate model for mentorship, guidance, teaching, and in today's world, coaching. In fact, the whole point of being an elder is to contribute to the welfare and survival of the tribe.

All of which may sound odd to our modern ears. In the corporate world, leadership is often taken to be nothing more than a form of professional advancement, another resume-building item that will propel one's career to the highest level. But as a Native American meme puts it, "Leadership isn't about advancing yourself. Leadership is about advancing your people." In fact, this mission is taken as a sacred obligation and an awesome responsibility in native communities. What better use of the elder's experience than to return it to the people?

The good news is that there's a powerful sense of meaning and purpose here, one that benefits both the tribe and the elders themselves. By giving our experience away in service, we expand our influence into the future and become stronger in the process. In fact, this meaning-inspired action is probably more clinically effective than many of the popular health practices that we hear so much about today.

But what of today's leaders, teachers, coaches, and activists? Conditions are murky and in one sense at least, far more complex and demanding than our ancestral experience on the grassland. Carnivores were bad enough, but what should we be teaching about today's ecosocial chaos? What path should the tribe take? What life lessons make sense in a world on the brink? And most importantly, how do we move people to new behaviors, attitudes, and deeper engagement?

In a way, modern teachers, coaches and activists are very much like the philosopher of Plato's cave. As you might remember, Plato imagined a group of people chained in a dark cave, watching as the light from a fire cast flickering shapes upon the wall. By appearance, the shadows seem to reveal the nature of the world, but in fact, they're only illusions. The philosopher and the activist are those who've escaped the cave and discovered the true—and sometimes disturbing—nature of reality on the outside.

Plato's allegory is a perfect metaphor for the digital addiction of our time, but it also implies a job description for the activist coach—pulling people out of distraction and into contact with the real, natural, life-giving world. In this sense, we might well say that teachers, coaches, and activists are really attentional therapists—leaders who help us see the world in new, more functional ways.

But leadership is about far more than content, information, and technique. If we're going to move people into new behaviors, it's not enough to simply show up and start talking. Lofty words and eloquence are all well and good, but it's authenticity and risk-taking that really inspire people to new perspectives and ways of living. As intensely social animals, we pay extremely close attention to the way our teachers, coaches, and elders actually live. Are they walking their talk? Are they playing it safe, or are they actually living in a way that's consistent with their beliefs? In the end, conviction, courage, and authenticity are the qualities that really get people's attention.

HOW WE SHOW UP

The years go by, and we discover that being an activist or artivist is not an easy path. We try to create change in our lives and the world, but we find that we're up against immense, wickedly complex, and highly dynamic systems: social systems, culture, big organizations, governments, not to mention the atmosphere and biological systems themselves. We touch the world with some intent, plot our actions, measure everything in sight and make our best guesses, but it's not always clear that we're having the desired effect, or even any effect at all. All of which might make us feel helpless, insignificant, and frustrated; we might even be inclined to throw up our hands and forget the whole thing.

The historian and philosopher Will Durant once observed that "education is the progressive discovery of our own ignorance." Or to put it another way, "education is the progressive discovery of our own powerlessness." With each passing year, the world is revealed to be far, far bigger and more complex than we had ever imagined and we might even begin to see ourselves as insignificant.

But it's important to remember that complex systems don't behave in linear, predictable ways. These systems are extremely sensitive to initial conditions, butterfly effects, ripples and cascades of influence. So while we can't really control or predict the specific outcome of our actions, we do have substantial control over something even more important: the way we show up.

In other words, we may not be able to exert pin-point control over particular issues, policies, programs or events, but if we engage with the right attitude, posture, and perspective, we *will* have a positive effect. You may not see it in your lifetime, but rest assured; showing up with integrity, dignity, sincerity, and respect *always* touches the world, even if you're not around to see the results.

All of which might not sound like much. As activists and artivists, want to be effective and we want results, especially in this age of urgency. Will showing up with dignity, integration, curiosity, and sincerity really move the needle on the world? We can never really know the ultimate consequences, but we do know this: showing up with sincerity and relevance is simply a better way to live.

In turn, this orientation calls us to re-examine our conventional, familiar notions of success and failure. We all know the standard narrative, as we've been conditioned to it almost from birth: Success comes through achievement, possession, and status. Accomplish great things, get a bunch of fancy stuff, surround yourself with fancy people and live a life of material and social affluence. And if you fail to achieve this, well then, better luck next time.

In the world of activism, the same conditioning leads us to similar conclusions and we're quick to pin our notions of success and failure on tangible victories and achievements. Push through some legislation, elect a better candidate, stop a fossil fuel project, or protect a bioregion from development—these successes make us feel good, feed our sense of accomplishment and give us the juice to carry on. If we fail in these efforts, we lose heart and might even drop out of the movement entirely. But given what we now know about the behavior of complex systems, this framing is not just wrong, it sets us up for unhappiness and even despair.

A better way is to put our focus, not on results and achievement, but on high-quality engagement, in other words, showing up with our best possible effort. This is precisely the approach advocated by legendary athletic coach John Wooden. As he saw it, showing up was everything. If you're showing up with your best game every day, there can be no failure. If you're practicing your art with sincerity and dignity, you've succeeded, full stop. In other words, doing your best—especially in these wickedly impossible circumstances—*is* success. Keep trying, even when it looks like you're going to lose. *Especially* when it looks like you're going to lose.

SUFFER WELL

> There can be no purpose more inspiring than
> to begin the age of restoration, reweaving the
> wondrous diversity of life that still surrounds us.
>
> E.O. Wilson

So we do our best. We keep showing up with a sense of artivism, martial artistry, and maybe even—on our good days—sapience. But the prognosis for humanity and the biosphere remains dark; conditions are deteriorating and the age of comfort is coming to an end. Millions of creatures—human and non-human alike—are suffering, with more to come. In our lifetimes, we're going to witness ecological and social disruption on a massive scale.

Radical change is now inevitable; in the coming months and years, we're going to be dragged out of our comfort zones and we have very little choice in the matter. Conditions will challenge us in a thousand ways, but there are things we can and must do…

Start by doing the inner work of adaptability, minimalism, and creative action. Learn some practical skills: gardening, home repair, water collection, and so on. Next, start getting comfortable with being uncomfortable. Exercise your courage and learn to accept a higher level of risk.

Along the way, all of us will have to get familiar with loss, tragedy, and senseless destruction of living things. This will not be easy. After all, many of us, especially in the affluent North, have come to expect, even demand, a secure, predictable, and controllable existence. Advertising fills our spirits with craving, desire, and promises of wonderful things that will come our way, but the reality is altogether different. In fact, everything we hold dear is going away. As the Buddhist writer Pico Iyer has put it, "loss is the law of life." Everything we've ever loved is temporary; our health, our loved ones, our familiar comforts, and yes, even the integrity of the biosphere.

So don't be surprised by your personal losses or our collective tragedies; this is part of the process. Fight the fight as skillfully as you can, but without expectation. Maintain your dignity, honesty, and integrity, even in the face of outrageous adversity. Ignore the haters and the inactivists, work where you are, create where you are. Ignore the defeats and keep your focus on the means, the path, the journey. Keep showing up with your best game, every day, no matter what. And remember, engagement *is* success.

GRATITUDE AND APPRECIATIONS

Activism may well be therapeutic and even medicinal, but it's not an easy life. Every day brings a new round of exposure, stress, and ambiguity, but that's just the beginning. We engage as best we can and fight the good fight, but we often feel a sense of isolation, loneliness, and alienation from the cultural mainstream; we stand unappreciated and sometimes even reviled on the fringe of society.

On some days it feels like we're surrounded by legions of dedicated inactivists, people who haven't yet had their encounter with The Knowledge, or having had the encounter, opted for disengagement and irrelevance. Content with their lives as is, they don't really give much thought to the future or the planet. Like dinosaurs on that fateful day some 65 million years ago, they aren't much inclined to look up, much less take up the fight.

To make matters worse, those around us are often quick to shoot the messenger; to discount, ignore or abuse anyone who speaks the inconvenient truths of our world. And on the rare occasions when we're actually listened to, we're dismissed out of hand as Cassandras (from Greek mythology, a Trojan priestess fated to utter true prophecies but never to be believed). Along the way, we also come to the disturbing realization that many people feel threatened and intimidated by our very existence. The mere presence of activism in the world implies that others aren't doing enough, aren't being enough. And no one wants a buzzkill at their party.

It's an eerie, exhausting sensation and on some days we might even wish we'd never bothered to become aware of our predicament in the first place. Ignorance might not actually be bliss, but it would be nice to feel culturally "normal" and included on occasion. Things might be easier to bear, for a while at least.

But sometimes we get lucky. Every now and then, we bump into the wise ones, people with their lights on, people who do their homework and live with a commitment to relevance and engagement. In my life, I've been radically fortunate to run into two such individuals: John Hagar and Jonathan Logan, kindred spirits and colleagues in Activism is Medicine, teachers and senseis both.

Powerful inspirations and support have also come my way from Rodney King, Corey Jung, Steve Myrland and Kellie Murphy, Guy McPherson, Michael Dowd, Louie and Gerlinde Gelina, Susan Fahringer, Jill Stephenson, Alessandro Pelizzon, Jeremy Lent, Paul Landon, Steve Laskevitch and Carla Fraga, Sebastien Alary and Anne Smith, Derrick Jensen, Max Wilbert, Skye Nacel, David Kopacz, Pete Karabetis, Michael Campi, Barb Moro and Diedre Knowlton, Dana Lyons, Amelia DuBose and all the youth climate activists in Bend, OR.

And most of all, the love of my life, Sue Schwantes.

Thank you all for keeping me whole.

ABOUT THE AUTHOR

Frank Forencich is a passionate advocate for the human animal and a functional future. He earned his BA at Stanford University in human biology and has over thirty years of teaching experience in martial art and health education.

Frank holds black belt rankings in karate and aikido and has traveled to Africa on several occasions to study human origins and the ancestral environment. He's presented at numerous venues, including the Ancestral Health Symposium, Google, the Dr. Robert D. Conn Heart Conference, the Welsh Pain Society, and the Stanford University Institute of Design. Frank is the author of numerous books about health and the human predicament and is a Diplomate member at The American Institute of Stress.

Contact Frank at humananimal.earth